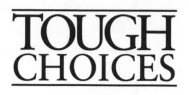

TOUGH
CHOICES

In the series Health, Society, and Policy,
edited by Sheryl Ruzek and Irving Kenneth Zola

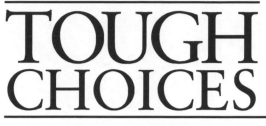

TOUGH
CHOICES

*In Vitro Fertilization
and the Reproductive Technologies*

■

Edited by
PATRICIA STEPHENSON
and
MARSDEN G. WAGNER

Temple University Press
Philadelphia

Temple University Press, Philadelphia 19122
Copyright © 1993 by Temple University. All rights reserved
Published 1993
Printed in the United States of America

Portions of the Introduction were published previously in *Social and Preventive Medicine* 1992;37:213–217 and are included here with the permission of Birkhäuser Publishers.

An earlier version of Chapter 6 was published in the *International Journal of Technology Assessment in Health Care* 1991;7:585–593. Material is reproduced here with the permission of Cambridge University Press.

An earlier version of Chapter 7 was published in *Iatrogenics* 1991;1:7–16. Material is reproduced here with the permission of Munksgaard.

An earlier version of Chapter 10 was published in the *European Journal of Public Health* 1991;1:45–50. Material is reproduced here with the permission of Scandinavian University Press.

An earlier version of Chapter 11 was published in the *International Journal of Health Sciences* 1991;2:119–123. Material is reproduced here with the permission of Van Gorcum.

The paper used in this publication meets the minimum requirements
of American National Standard for Information Sciences—Permanence
of Paper for Printed Library Materials, ANSI Z39.48-1984 ⊗

Library of Congress Cataloging-in-Publication Data

Tough choices : in vitro fertilization and the reproductive
    technologies / edited by Patricia Stephenson and Marsden G. Wagner.
        p.   cm. — (Health, society, and policy)
    ISBN 1-56639-060-5 (alk. paper)
    1. Human reproductive technology—Social aspects.   2. Infertility-
-Treatment—Technological innovations—Social aspects.
    3. Fertilization in vitro, Human—Social aspects.   I. Stephenson,
Patricia, 1954–   .   II. Wagner, Marsden, 1930–   .   III. Series.
    [DNLM: 1. Fertilization in Vitro—methods.   2. Reproduction
Techniques.   WQ 205 T722]
RG133.5.T68   1993
362.1'96692—dc20   92-48989

CONTENTS

PART III   RISK ASSESSMENT

PART IV   LAW AND ETHICS

PREFACE

In vitro fertilization (IVF), gamete intrafallopian transfer (GIFT), zygote intrafallopian transfer (ZIFT), and related procedures are technologies (tools) intended to make life better. In and of themselves, technologies are neither "good" nor "evil." The application of technology can be said to be "appropriate" or "inappropriate." For example, a vacuum cleaner is handy in that it saves having to beat carpets and sweep floors; if one should use the vacuum cleaner to terrorize the family cat, however, then the technology has been applied in an inappropriate way that can cause the cat a great deal of physical and psychological harm. Perhaps this is overstating the point, but it should be acknowledged that medical technologies can, and often are, either overused or misused in practice.

To determine what is and is not an appropriate application of medical technology, information is required on the effectiveness, safety, costs, and benefits of the technology in question. Most governments in the industrialized world have developed elaborate systems for evaluating drugs before their introduction on the market, but not for medical technologies. Thus, more often than not the consumer receiving treatment also serves as a research subject while the health-care industry develops, modifies, and perfects medical technologies. This situation is largely unavoidable, but the medical field, industry, and government should at least attempt to build a thorough evaluation, using scientifically acceptable methods, into the process before widespread acceptance and application of technology. (Even vacuum cleaners must meet certain safety codes, in many countries, before patenting and marketing.)

Sadly, this type of evaluation is only just beginning for the so-called "new reproductive technologies" (IVF, GIFT, ZIFT, and so on), despite the fact that these technologies are now in widespread use. Their true value has not been determined, nor have the risks associated with such treatment been assessed adequately. Virtually no attempt has been made to determine the need for services in specific populations or the effectiveness of IVF and GIFT compared with other technologies designed to restore fertility. Little attention has been paid to preventing infertility in the first place or to the costs of treating infertility, both for individuals and society. Most importantly, there has been no concerted effort to examine the problem of infertility in the community and what governments and their policy makers should do about it.

Today, policy makers are beginning to ask these questions. Reports on the ethical, legal, regulatory, and funding aspects of IVF and GIFT as well as related technologies have been issued by governmental or nongovernmental bodies in Australia, Canada, Denmark, Germany, France, Israel, Italy, South Africa, Sweden, the United Kingdom, and the United States. Many other countries have had and are having considerable professional or public discussion concerning the new reproductive technologies.

Health-policy decisions involve tough choices, and these decisions must be informed by adequate data that have been analyzed with standard epidemiological methods and presented in a balanced manner. The participants in discussions concerning the application of these technologies must include, but should not be limited to, IVF and GIFT clinicians, pediatricians, epidemiologists, health services researchers, ethicists, legal experts, policy makers, social scientists, economists, people with infertility, and the public at large.

This book was written by and for professionals of the aforementioned disciplines, but it also is intended to be useful for infertile people and the general public. In the chapters that follow, we and the other authors discuss medical and social options for infertility; the effectiveness, safety, costs, and benefits of the new reproductive technologies; and some legal and ethical issues surrounding use of these services.

Our purpose is not to challenge the existence of the new reproductive technologies from a moral or ethical standpoint, or to debate the rights of eggs and embryos. We acknowledge from the very beginning that these technologies are in use, that people want them, and that they will continue to be available in health care systems. Our concern is the appropriate use of the new reproductive technologies in health systems and in infertility care.

Patricia Stephenson
Marsden G. Wagner

Karlstad, Sweden

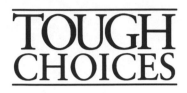

TOUGH
CHOICES

INTRODUCTION

Infertility and In Vitro Fertilization: Is the Tail Wagging the Dog?

■

MARSDEN G. WAGNER *and* PATRICIA STEPHENSON

> *The greatest danger arises from ruthless application of partial knowledge on a vast scale.*
> —E. F. SCHUMACHER

Today, national commissions and parliamentary committees in nearly every industrialized country are struggling to resolve many contentious issues concerning the new reproductive technologies. There is a lack of scientifically valid information derived from clinical trials and other epidemiological studies. Also lacking are assessments of benefits and costs, studies of the social consequences of infertility treatment, and discussions of ethical issues. The absence of this information stymies governmental efforts to formulate public policy on infertility and its treatment with IVF, GIFT, and other related technologies. No new technology should be widely diffused or integrated as accepted medical management until such a scientific assessment has been completed.[1] We believe that until the data are in, a new technology must remain an experimental procedure and its use be guided by all the principles and safeguards covering research on human subjects. This, however, is not the current state of affairs.

Governments, doctors, and the public do not fully appreciate the experimental nature of the new reproductive technologies. Despite this, a serious problem of uncontrolled proliferation exists. It is estimated that more than 700 IVF programs are in place in 53 countries.[2] Over 100,000 treatment cycles have been performed and 5,000 babies born in the decade after the first IVF birth.[3] In several countries, the pace at which services have expanded has been truly astonishing; Israel, for example, a country of 4.4 million people, has 18 IVF programs.[2] The Netherlands has 12 programs and 30 affiliated satellite clinics to serve a population of 15 million.[4] Australia has 22 programs to serve a population of 16.7 million,[5] and France, a country of 56 million people, supports approximately 80 officially recognized and an unknown number of unrecognized programs.[6] Even India, a country where enormous human and monetary resources have been applied toward controlling population growth, now officially encourages IVF as a treatment for infertility; many private clinics (usually franchises from industrialized countries) and government-run facilities offer the procedure.[7]

Such rapid proliferation of services could not have occurred without an ever-increasing pool of eligible candidates for treatment; an expanded list of indications for IVF supported this proliferation. From its beginnings as a treatment for women with damaged fallopian tubes, IVF came to be regarded as suitable treatment for infertility caused by endometriosis, ovulation disorders, antisperm antibodies, genital tract tuberculosis, diethylstilbestrol-associated cervical abnormalities, and idiopathic infertility.[8] More recently, indications for IVF have been extended to include male factors,[9] thereby exposing women to the risks associated with IVF procedures because of their partners' condition.

Moreover, the adoption of broad but rigid definitions of infertility, uninformed by a thorough understanding of the normal variation in fecundity and the natural history of infertility, led to spuriously inflated estimates of the prevalence of infertility. Infertility has become a kind of new morbidity—a medical reconstruction of a social problem, that is, involuntary childlessness. Medicalization brings with it an emphasis on medical and technological solutions.

Media descriptions and popular sources give the public the impression that there is an epidemic of infertility. Proponents of IVF state that the prevalence of infertility in the community is approximately 10% to 20%. It has been suggested by some that one out of six couples is infertile and that the problem is growing worse. But what is the validity of, and scientific basis for, these statements? In the following sections, we discuss the prevalence and etiology of infertility as well as the relevance of this information for national infertility services and prevention programs.

PREVALENCE OF INFERTILITY

Prevalence estimates are affected by the criteria used for making the diagnosis of the particular condition in question. A clear, agreed-on, measurable definition is needed to diagnose people as either having or not having the condition. The better the definition, the lower the probability that a person will be misdiagnosed.

Some conditions are easy to diagnose. For example, a simple test can determine whether a woman's blood type is Rh (rhesus) negative or not. Unfortunately, infertility is not so easy to diagnose because the ability to conceive is a continuum ranging from absolute sterility through subfertility to normal fertility and, perhaps, even superfertility. The cut-off point on the continuum, where normal is differentiated from abnormal, is entirely arbitrary. There is no agreed-on standard definition of infertility. Even two such august bodies as the World Health Organization (WHO) and the United States Office of Technology Assessment (OTA) cannot agree. WHO defines infertility as not conceiving after cohabitation and exposure to the possibility of pregnancy for two years,[10] while the OTA definition is the inability to conceive after 12 months of intercourse without contraception.[7]

Both definitions are inherently flawed; they allow a substantial proportion of normal, fertile people to be misdiagnosed as infertile. When the definition of 12 months of unprotected intercourse is used, only 16% to 21% of couples meeting this definition actually remain infertile throughout their lives.[7] Indeed, several studies suggest that about 30% of couples take more than a year to conceive at some time during their reproductive lives.[11,12]

A reassessment of data from the World Fertility Survey and other studies does not substantiate a core rate of infertility of 10% to 20%.[13] A survey in the United States reported that 8.5% of married couples with the wife aged 15 to 44 years ($n = 8,450$) were infertile,[14] an estimate that is undoubtedly too high as an indicator of actual lifetime infertility as the OTA definition of infertility was used. Only 3.8% of that sample had *never* given birth, whereas 4.7% had one or more births before the onset of infertility.[14] These figures obtained in 1988 were unchanged from a previous survey conducted in 1982.[14]

ETIOLOGY OF INFERTILITY

The causes of infertility are many and varied. The WHO Task Force Standardized Investigation of the Infertile Couple[15,16] is the largest study of infertility ever conducted. More than 10,000 couples in 25 countries have been enrolled in the study,[16] and the published 1985 results ($n = 8,450$) show that tubal obstruction or pelvic adhesion are the most common causes of infertility in the female, accounting for approximately 24% of all female infertility in developed countries.[16] Other specific diagnoses for the underlying cause of female infertility are: no demonstrable cause, 40%; acquired tubal abnormality, 12%; anovulatory regular cycles, 10%; anovulatory oligomenorrhea, 9%; ovulatory oligomenorrhea, 7%; hyperprolactinemia, 7%; and endometriosis, 6%. In the male partner the specific diagnoses are: no demonstrable cause, 49%; varicocele, 11%; primary idiopathic testicular failure, 10% accessory gland infection, 7%; abnormal sperm morphology, 8%; and low sperm motility, 3%. (Not all diagnoses are listed; subjects also may have more than one diagnosis.)

The presence of tubal obstruction or pelvic adhesions usually indicates previous pelvic inflammatory disease (PID).[15] PID (symptomatic or asymptomatic) usually is caused by sexually transmitted diseases, especially *Chlamydia trachomatis* and gonorrhea.[15] PID also may occur after induced abortion, birth, surgery, intrauterine device (IUD) insertion, or other invasive procedures.[15]

In turn, PID is associated with infertility. In a Swedish study of 15- to 24-year-old women, one episode of PID was associated with infertility in 9.4% of cases, two episodes in 20.9%, and three or more episodes in 51.6%.[17] Studies in Sweden and the United States show that postabortion PID is 3 to 30 times higher in women with untreated *Chlamydia* cervical infection than in treated women.[18,19] Another study demonstrated that 40% of post-abortal women infected with *Chlamydia* will develop PID,[20] and when induced abortion is illegally performed, PID rates are likely higher. Infection with *Chlamydia* is increasingly common in pregnant women who do not abort, and approximately 25% of infected pregnant women develop intrapartum fever or postpartum endometritis.[21]

According to the aforementioned WHO study, a history of postabortion or postpartum infection carries a relative risk of 4.2 (95% CI, 2.9 to 6.6) for bilateral tubal occlusion.[17] In developed countries, 24% of women with bilateral tubal occlusion had a history of postabortion or postpartum infection, and 28% had a history of sexually transmitted disease.[23] The male equivalent of tubal obstruction following infection is the blocking of the vasa differentia and chronic infection of accessory glands. The reason for the low rate of infection-related infertility in men is unknown. The male however, plays a significant role in the causation of infection-related female infertility; approximately 90% of female partners of men with gonorrhea and 60% of female partners of men with *Chlamydia* will become infected.[22] More importantly, infection-related infertility in the female is associated with a positive history of infection in the male partner. When WHO investigators analyzed data from all subjects for whom a diagnosis was reached in the female partner and used those women with infection-related diagnoses but no history of infection in either partner as the reference group, the relative risk of infertility increased 56% when the male partner had a positive history of infection, 82% when the female partner had a positive history, and 124% when both partners had positive histories.[16]

In addition to the causes noted, a number of surgical procedures are associated with infertility. These include tubal sterilization, vasectomy, ovarian wedge resection, appendectomy, uterine suspension, cesarean section, hysterosalpingography, infant hernia repair, and dilatation and curettage.[7] While some of these procedures are quite common, no data exists on their contribution to overall rates of infertility.

Some drugs may affect fertility as well. Diethystilbestrol (DES) has been associated with infertility in both sons and daughters of women who took the drug while pregnant.[7] Overprescription or incorrect prescription of fertility drugs also can cause hyperstimulation and infertility.[7]

Other social, psychological, and lifestyle factors are associated with infertility. Excessive strenuous exercise, rapid weight loss, low body fat, stress, smoking, and long-term alcohol consumption reduce fertility, as does exposure to certain environmental toxins in the workplace.[7] Many acute or chronic illnesses can cause anovulation or decreased spermatogenesis,[7] and whether a couple conceives within a given time also is influenced strongly by the frequency of intercourse. In one study, 16.7% of couples having intercourse less than once a week conceived within 6 months, but 83.3% of couples having intercourse four or more times a week conceived within that same period.[24]

POLICY IMPLICATIONS OF DEFINITIONS OF INFERTILITY

These data indicate that the true prevalence of infertility in the community is far below 10% to 20%. While it is true that perhaps 8% of couples may, at some point, have difficulty conceiving, only a fraction actually remain childless. One then may infer that the accepted clinical definition of infertility (12 months of unprotected intercourse) inevitably results in overdiagnosis and that overtreatment unnecessarily exposes women to the risks associated with drugs and invasive procedures. Of course, the impact of unnecessary medical care on national health budgets is staggering.

Estimates of the need for infertility treatment services, therefore, must be based on conservative estimates of prevalence. For clinical practice and health service–planning needs, a definition of 2 years of exposure to the risk of pregnancy is most appropriate.

Today, the medical community pressures health policy makers to label IVF as the standard treatment for infertility. Indeed, it is standard in a number of countries and often reimbursed by public funds meant for general health services. Nevertheless, many scientists and ethicists argue that the new reproductive technologies must still be considered experimental given the paucity of data on their safety, effectiveness, and cost-effectiveness.[25]

The rapid, widespread proliferation of IVF is not justified by its scientific assessment. Despite favorable reports in the professional and lay press, published prospective, randomized, controlled experimental trials to ascertain the efficacy and risks of IVF are lacking.[26] (One such trial is in progress, but results are not yet available.)[27] Almost all medical articles on IVF are nonevaluative descriptions and uncontrolled comparisons of procedures. Current research focuses on perfecting the clinical details in the various steps of IVF, not on assessing outcomes.

The effort to assess IVF scientifically has been seriously hampered by the lack of sound, uniform, population-based data. Findings usually are reported using single-clinic populations. The few surveys that have been done, with the exception of those in Australia/New Zealand and the United Kingdom, are of little or no value, because the clinics voluntarily decide whether to participate.

MEASURING "SUCCESS"

As a result of inadequately controlled, population-based data on IVF, great confusion exists concerning its true efficacy. Moreover, different measures of success are applied. But how is efficacy or success measured? Doctors have defined success as pregnancy. The infertile woman's goal is a healthy baby, and for her, a successful outcome is a live birth or preferably a "take-home" baby. Because of the high incidence of pregnancy loss after IVF, however, these two success rates are quite different.

Clinicians found they could increase the chance for a pregnancy by hyperstimulating the ovaries and then transferring multiple eggs or embryos. Later, scientists showed that such practices markedly increased multiple birth rates, low-birth-weight rates, and both perinatal and neonatal mortality rates. Redefining success as a healthy baby casts a different light on hyperstimulation and multiple egg or embryo transfer, and a few clinicians are now considering a return to IVF using a woman's natural cycle.[26] Others advocate freezing eggs or embryos for sequential tries or for donation.

Recently, it has become popular to report cumulative success rates, for example, the percentage of women who achieve a pregnancy or a live birth within three cycles of treatment. Reporting success in this way can have certain advantages, but care must be taken not to confuse success rates calculated on the basis of a single treatment with cumulative rates that are much more optimistic. In addition, cumulative success rates are not accompanied by cumulative risk rates and costs during most discussions with policymakers or the public.

WHAT ARE THE RISKS?

As the focus of clinical research on IVF has been improving efficacy, there is an alarming lack of epidemiologic studies of risks associated with treatment of women and their children. Even descriptive articles related to risk are few and far between, despite the medical maxim, "first do no harm." To adequately determine the psychological as well as physical risks to the woman and to the baby, both must be monitored for years after treatment. Such follow-up has been hindered by the fragmented nature of reproductive health services; when a woman receiving IVF succeeds in becoming pregnant, she usually is referred elsewhere for pregnancy and birth care. Information on the progress of her pregnancy, complications, and the fate of the fetus or infant often are not reported to the IVF-treatment provider. As Blyth states: "With few exceptions the debate over the last few years has taken little account of the interests of the children to be created by the assisted reproduction techniques. Considerably more effort has gone into questioning the morality of storing and experimenting with embryos up to two weeks old than on the future prospects of live children."[28]

No country in the world has an effective system to guarantee that diffusion of a new technology will not occur before its risks are determined. Most have a system that prohibits the marketing of new drugs until an initial assessment of risk has been carried out, but once a new drug is on the market, licensed physicians are free to use that drug as they see fit. Thus, while the drugs used in IVF have been approved for use at certain dosages under certain conditions, the risks (particularly the long-term risks) associated with their repeated use in higher doses and in combination with other drugs during IVF have not been determined, nor have the psychological risks been explored.

WHAT ARE THE COSTS?

The costs of IVF are generally underestimated. To be calculated correctly, the cost to society per liveborn IVF baby must include not only the direct costs of the IVF procedures used in one successful case but also the costs of the failures. Furthermore, valid estimates of financial costs must include the cost of all the documented, subsequent medical procedures found more frequently in IVF pregnancies, including hospitalization during pregnancy, cesarean section and other interventions during birth, and referrals for neonatal intensive care. Calculated this way, the costs to society for one healthy IVF baby far exceed the estimates given in the clinical literature.

Where does this money come from? In countries with a large

private health sector, IVF has become a lucrative enterprise. One study estimates the IVF private market in the United States at $30 to $40 million per year.[29] In private medical care, this means that IVF is an option for the wealthy or for those willing to commit their life savings. On the other hand, when government subsidies cover some or all IVF-treatment charges, the cost to the public is enormous. In countries such as Australia and Israel, taxpayers are paying for this costly technology that benefits only a few. The public also pays for the hidden costs of IVF; nearly all physicians working in IVF clinics (public or private) received their medical and postgraduate training courtesy of the taxpayers and may have received training in institutions supported by public funds.

WHO BENEFITS FROM FERTILITY MANAGEMENT STRATEGIES?

Nevertheless, the public is usually happy to foot the bill so long as there are decided benefits to be gained from the use of medical technology. For the couple with a healthy baby resulting from IVF, and for the clinicians who assist them, the benefit is enormous. But decision makers must balance such benefits to selected individuals against the overall, limited benefits of IVF to society.[30] In other words, the perspective must shift from the individual focus of the clinical model to the group approach of the public health model, which asks the question: What is the contribution of IVF to the reduction of infertility in the community?

In considering the benefits of IVF from this new perspective, it is essential that the starting point be all infertile people in the community and the end point be a wanted, healthy baby (Figure 1). Infertile people have options, and it is they who choose what they want while service providers assist them in this choice from time to time. Furthermore, IVF is but one option among other medical and social options. The recent emphasis on IVF has tended to obscure the importance of these other possibilities.

Figure 1 also illustrates what some have called the roller-coaster character of IVF procedures.[8,29] When a step in the process

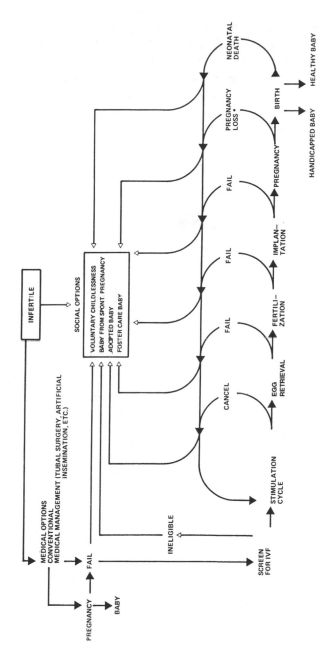

Figure 1. Options for infertile people.

* INCLUDING SPONTANEOUS ABORTION, ECTOPIC PREGNANCY, FETAL DEATH.

succeeds, an emotional high occurs. However, when a step fails, there is an emotional low as well as the need for the woman to decide to start the stimulation cycle over again or to move to social options. In a survey of Dutch women, a majority reported that the stress of waiting to see if they were pregnant was the most unpleasant part of the process.[31] In an Australian study, the second most common reason for dropping out after one failed attempt (finance being the most common) was the stress, anxiety, and pressure.[32]

Figure 2 attempts to represent, albeit in a nonquantitative

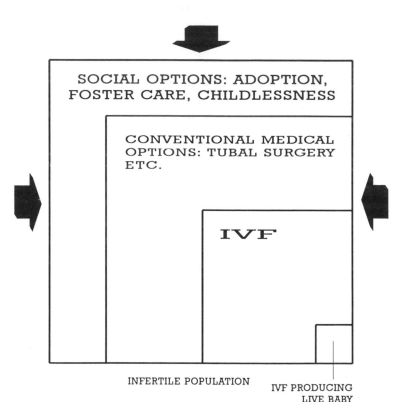

Figure 2. Contributions of in vitro fertilization to the infertile population. Arrows indicate effect of preventive programs to reduce the infertile population.

manner, the place of IVF in overall infertility care. The place of infertility prevention has been markedly neglected. Workers in IVF clinics express concern for individual women to conceive, but there is little evidence that this extrapolates to a concern for overall infertility in the community and its prevention. In the medical literature, an article on the prevention of infertility is rare. WHO recommends that priority be given to prevention and primary care, which is not today's approach to infertility. For the cost of one live IVF baby, it is likely that many women could be prevented from ever becoming infertile in the first place through programs to prevent sexually transmitted diseases, health education, and infectious disease control methods.[33]

PREVENTION

A review of what is known about the causes of infertility and the potential for prevention does not support the nihilistic attitude of IVF proponents toward prevention. In a rational plan for the overall management of infertility in the community, prevention must come first. Such efforts benefit the whole community, not just a few individuals, and good evidence supports the redirection of research priorities, health manpower resources, and health care expenditures away from high-tech medical treatment and toward infertility prevention programs.

Because approximately one-third of all infertility is caused by potentially preventable infections, renewed efforts to control sexually transmitted diseases are required as well. Sexually transmitted disease prevention and control programs also can help reduce pregnancy wastage, cervical malignancy, and the transmission of the human immunodeficiency virus (HIV).

Low-cost, mass-screening technology for *Chlamydia* and other sexually transmitted diseases is available. Antibiotic treatment of infected individuals is safe and effective. Higher priority should go to health education for the public (including schoolchildren), improved detection and treatment of disease, better education of health professionals, and contact tracing. Contact tracing would be facilitated by making *Chlamydia* infection and its symptoms (nonspecific urethritis in the male) reportable; at the moment, Sweden is the only country where *Chlamydia* infection is a notifiable disease.

Iatrogenic causes of infertility also are preventable. These include surgeries, invasive diagnostic procedures, drugs, and unrecognized and untreated infections. Prevention efforts in this area must be directed toward health professionals. Educating physicians to the risks posed by abdominal surgery (including cesarean section) to future fertility is one means of preventing iatrogenic infertility. Education can point out, for example, the potential harm done to women by unnecessary cesarean sections and frequent vaginal examinations during labor. Education programs also can stress the importance of aggressive management of PID and conservative treatment that avoids pelvic surgery and other invasive procedures in young women. Proper screening for and treatment of sexually transmitted disease during pregnancy and before abortion can go a long way toward preventing infertility. Also, surgical sterilization techniques in women should minimize the damage done to the fallopian tubes in case the woman should ever seek reversal of the procedure.

More research is needed to determine the causes of male infertility and how it might be prevented. Programs for the prevention and treatment of infertility inevitably direct their efforts to women, and research programs do the same. Prevention of male infertility is neglected despite strong evidence that men and women make a nearly equal contribution to the pathogenesis of infertility.

More research is needed on psychosomatic and social factors of infertility. That no cause of infertility could be found in a significant number of couples in the WHO study may simply indicate that unrecognized, biological factors were present, but it also may indicate that psychosomatic factors have a presently undefined role in the etiology of infertility.

Lastly, more research is needed on the appropriate use of medical technology and quality assurance in health care. Directly or indirectly, invasive medical procedures can render a woman infertile. Little data exists on the contribution of iatrogenesis to overall infertility, but there is good reason to believe this is significant. Research is needed on how to change physician practices, because education may not be enough. Research is needed on quality assurance strategies to reduce the number of unnecessary invasive interventions and their harmful consequences.

WHAT ARE THE ALTERNATIVES?

As an editorial pointed out, "Resources and attention are being diverted from prevention of infertility and from acquisition of primary obstetric skills to being able to see, monitor and intervene with ultrasound, hormonal assays and surgery in ever more minute steps in (artificial) reproduction. Professional attention is diverted from caring for patients to developing increasingly narrow ranges of technical skills."[34] When the focus of infertility services is on IVF, there are subtle influences on skills and attitudes, a tilting of the health manpower balance away from prevention and caring toward searching for technological solutions and clinical treatment.[34] The result is a serious diversion of financial and human resources away from community health needs, ironically sapping resources away from overall infertility management.

Figure 2 illustrates how only a small number of the overall infertile population can be expected to have a healthy baby through IVF. There are no figures available on what proportion of the infertile population chooses social options, nor any data on the proportion choosing conventional medical options or IVF. We do, however, have some information on the proportion of those choosing IVF who will bring home a baby.

Not all infertile women are candidates for IVF. Some will be screened out during the selection process, and an additional 20% to 25% will fail the early steps of the procedure and drop out before embryo transfer. Reliable figures are hard to obtain, but if we take the most optimistic scenario, then perhaps 60% of all infertile women choosing IVF are theoretically capable of benefiting from it. These women will pass the selection process, succeed at the early steps, and reach the embryo-transfer stage. Because the best reported pregnancy rates following embryo transfer are between 20% and 40% however, then optimistically, only 30% of the original 60% (or 18% of all women who seek treatment) will become pregnant, and one-third to one-half of these pregnancies will result in fetal death and not produce a live birth. Therefore, the optimal figure theoretically possible from maximum use even of the most skilled IVF providers is 10% to 12% live-births per treatment cycle among all infertile women choosing this option.

Using up to three cycles of treatment on each woman eligible for and choosing IVF could then result, in a most optimistic figure, of 25% having a live-birth. Not all infertile women and men seek IVF, however. Many choose social options (adoption or childlessness) or another type of medical option. If we assume that 50% of infertile women will choose social or other medical options, then the proportion of all infertile women who theoretically could have a live baby from IVF is 12.5%. This figure has practical significance for health policy makers.

NEGLECTED ISSUES

Because of the lack of a public health approach to IVF, far too little attention has been given to the important social, ethical, and legal issues. The complexity of these issues prohibits detailed discussion here, but several general points should be made. First, these issues tend to be defined too narrowly, limited to issues surrounding the details of IVF procedures. For example, the banking of spare human embryos raises many ethical and legal problems about storing human life, questions about what to do if the parents die, disagreements about disposition of embryos never reclaimed, and so on. These are urgent and important issues, but they affect only that small group of women who get to the embryo-transfer stage. Other issues affect much larger groups of people yet receive little or no attention: Should there be any social criteria for IVF recipients? Does society have a responsibility to deal with the long-term consequences of the technology? What is to be done about the diversion of money, resources, and health professionals' talents away from pressing community health needs into a high-tech procedure benefiting only a few? What are the best ways to handle ethically questionable clinical practices such as inducements to women to donate their eggs to IVF clinics and misrepresentation of success rates?

Second, complex social, legal, and ethical issues tend to be managed too narrowly by interest groups. Not only have service providers themselves failed to reach a consensus on policies, procedures, and ethical stances, but the officially designated groups established to address these issues (hospital ethical committees, regulatory agencies, and so on) are dominated by health professionals who have a vital interest in the outcome. These health professionals sometimes choose the lawyers and "ethicists" who also serve on these groups.[28]

Ownership of the information on IVF is another neglected issue. Appropriate use of technology includes the principle of fully informed choice by the individual user; in the case of IVF, an experimental procedure, the information base is inadequate. Women are unlikely to get sufficiently extensive and adequate information. One study that interviewed women who had tried IVF revealed "the need to investigate the way this technology is marketed, particularly the way success rates are calculated and communicated to patients, the way hospitals sell experimental procedures to patients, and the way physicians disclose the risks and disappointing possibilities during attempts at in vitro fertilization."[35] A particular concern to women who have experienced IVF was the way success rates were communicated to them: "staff members referred to 20–25% pregnancy rates, but failed to add that around 40% of women never reached the stage of embryo transfer from which the rates are calculated. Women who found out about high cancellations only after entering the program reported surprise and disappointment."[35]

Equally important, adequate information is essential to policy makers. Media coverage of IVF has tended toward sensationalism, with continual reports of "breakthroughs" and a focus on the most controversial ethical issues. False claims also cloud the true benefits. Together with the claims about success, all of this publicity has led both the general public and health professionals to hold a distorted view of the benefits of IVF and its place in infertility services.

TOWARD PUBLIC POLICY-MAKING

The problems associated with IVF (including proliferation; efficacy; risks; cost; benefit; and social, ethical, and legal issues) are compounded by a lack of direction and monitoring. No country has yet developed a rational plan for managing infertility or an adequate system of quality assurance. Perhaps one reason for the lack of public policy development on IVF is the reluctance of public officials to confront the volatile issues of women's rights, religion, and sexuality in the public debate.

The methodology is available for rational infertility planning at national, regional, and local levels. Infertility prevalence can be reliably estimated. The availability and use of social and medical options can be surveyed. The efficacy of various options can be calculated if the service providers cooperate fully. Information on medical and social-psychological risk can be gathered. Overall cost of the options can be estimated, and the general public can be surveyed regarding appropriate priorities for the infertility options as well as the priority of infertility vis-à-vis other social and health problems.

Using mass media and other methods, this information can be disseminated to the public as well as policy makers to help societies move toward establishing some consensus on the benefits of various options in fertility management and assigning priority for using societal resources to meet desired goals. Governments in several countries have initiated the development of public policy for IVF and other new reproductive technologies. More recent, extensive data on IVF, together with a broader mandate to include the overall management of all infertility, will move this effort forward toward rational planning of infertility services.

Along with a rational plan, every country also needs a system of quality assurance for the various options available to infertile people. This is particularly urgent in the case of IVF, because information on services has not always been reliable and the social, ethical, and legal issues are of such a serious nature. Such assurances include: setting standards of practice and identifying appropriate measurements, mandatory monitoring of the practices by an agency not involved in providing the same service, reporting of evaluations so that quality data are available to users of the services as well as the public and policy makers, and sanctioning of providers who do not meet standards of practice agreed upon by public bodies.

Standards of practice have been drawn up in several countries. In most cases, these standards are drafted by an organization of IVF clinicians concerned about the wide variation in the quality of services. This is an important start, but such peer standards tend to be general rather than specific, making it difficult to identify measures of quality. In a few cases, the government has collaborated in drafting the standards or the clinicians have invited outsiders, such as lawyers and ethicists, to participate. These tactics address a serious weakness of peer review (i.e., "the fox guarding the chickens" without any outsiders looking at what is going on).

With regard to the monitoring of IVF practices, several countries have created systems of reporting practices. When reporting is voluntary, those most in need of monitoring tend to be the least likely to report. The United Kingdom, for example, had a voluntary licensing authority for IVF, but after several years, a law was passed requiring reports to the government. Mandatory reporting cannot ensure the validity of the information provided, and for this reason, quality assurance also must require periodic, independent audits of individual clinics.

Information on the practices of individual clinics should be available to infertile individuals and the public. Australia has a good system of reporting from IVF clinics, but the information does not identify the individual clinics. Its data show a six-fold variation among IVF clinics regarding their efficacy, but infertile people in Australia cannot use this information in choosing clinics. In the United States, the organization of IVF clinicians gathered information from a large number of IVF clinics that elected to participate, but they published only aggregate rather than clinic-by-clinic data. Recognizing the need for specific data, a U.S. Congressman conducted a similar survey of practices and published the clinic-by-clinic results in the Congressional Record, allowing the information to be used by those seeking IVF services. However, few people read the Congressional Record or are likely to know that such information has been published; the legislator addressed the immediate problem but did not provide a permanent solution.

Finally, quality assurance must include sanctions against those failing to meet standards of practice. In the United States today, the reporting of information by IVF clinics is voluntary; there are no sanctions for not reporting and no sanctions for reporting substandard practices—a system that permits only partial quality assessment and not quality assurance. The new system in the United Kingdom, however, provides quality assurance. It requires government licensing of all IVF clinics, and licenses may be revoked.

Other governments are considering legislation for both the rational planning of services for infertility and quality assurance for the new reproductive technologies. We hope that the governments, in formulating such public policy, will be informed by interested parties (including the general public) and that they will draw on the experience of others as well as the principles of appropriate technology.

REFERENCES

1. World Health Organization, European Regional Office. Targets for Health for All. Copenhagen: Regional Office for Europe, WHO, 1986.
2. Schenker JG. Medically assisted conception. The state of the art in clinical practice. Background paper for the WHO-EURO Consulta-

tion on the Place of In Vitro Fertilization in Infertility Care, June 1990.

3. Banta HD. Technology assessment and in vitro fertilization. Background paper for the WHO-EURO Consultation on the Place of In Vitro Fertilization in Infertility Care, June 1990.

4. Haan G. Health services for infertility. Where does IVF fit in? Background paper for the WHO-EURO Consultation on the Place of In Vitro Fertilization in Infertility Care, June 1990.

5. Lancaster PAL. Assisted conception: health services and evaluation. Int J Technol Assess Health Care 1991;7:485–499.

6. Relier JP, Couchard M, Huon C. Risks of IVF: the neonatology experience. Background paper for the WHO-EURO Consultation on the Place of In Vitro Fertilization in Infertility Care, June 1990.

7. Congress of the United States, Office of Technology Assessment. Infertility: Medical Social Choices. Washington D.C.: U.S. Government Printing Office, 1988.

8. Holmes HB. In vitro fertilization, reflections on the state of the art. Birth 1988;15:134–144.

9. Acosta A, Chillik CF, Brugo S, et al. In vitro fertilization and the male factor. Urology 1986;28:1–9.

10. World Health Organization. The Epidemiology of Infertility: Report of a WHO Scientific Group. Geneva: WHO Technical Report Series no. 582, 1975.

11. Marchbanks PA, Peterson HB, Rubin GL, Cancer and Steroid Hormone Study Group. Research on infertility: definition makes a difference. Am J Epidemiol 1989;130:259–267.

12. Page H. Estimation of the prevalence and incidence of infertility in a population. Fertil Steril 1989;51:571–577.

13. Belsey MA. Infertility: prevalence, etiology and natural history. In: Brachman M, ed. Epidemiology of Perinatal Disorders. New Haven: Yale University Press, 1988: 255–281.

14. Mosher, WD, Pratt WF. Fecundity and infertility in the United States, 1965–88. Advance Data From Vital and Health Statistics. 1990;192:1–8.

15. Farley T. The WHO standardized investigation of the infertile couple. In: Ratman S, Teak E, Anandakuman C, eds. Infertility: Male and Female. Adv Fertil Steril 1987;4:7–19.

16. Progress: Newsletter of the Special Programme of Research, Development and Research Training in Human Reproduction 1990;15: 1–8.

17. Weström L. Incidence, prevalence and trends of acute pelvic inflammatory disease and its consequences in industrialized countries. Am J Obstet Gynecol 1980;138:880–892.

18. Westergaard L, Philipsen T, Sheibel J. Significance of cervical *Chlamydia* in postabortal PID. Obstet Gynecol 1982;60:322–325.
19. Osser S, Persson K. Post-abortal pelvic infection and the influence of humoral immunity. Am J Obstet Gynecol 1984;150:699–703.
20. Brunham RC, Peelin R, Maclean F, et al. Post-abortal C. *trachomatis* salpingitis correlating risk with antigen specific serologic responses and with neutralization. J Infect Dis 1987; 155:749–755.
21. Schacter J. Chlamydial infection in infants and its prevention. In: Mushahwar IK, ed. Sexually Transmitted Diseases: A Centennial Perspective. Chicago: Abbott Diagnostics, 1988:11–13.
22. WHO Task Force on the Diagnosis and Treatment of Infertility. Infections, pregnancies and infertility: perspectives on prevention. Fertil Steril 1987;47:964–968.
23. McGregor J, French J, Spenser N. Prevention of sexually transmitted disease in women. J Reprod Med 1988;33(suppl):109–118.
24. MacLeod J, Gold RZ. Cited in Behrman SJ, Kistner RW. Progress in Infertility, 2nd ed. Boston: Little Brown, 1975.
25. Caplan A. Arguing with success: is in vitro fertilization research or therapy? In: Beyond Baby M: Ethical Issues in New Reproductive Techniques. Clifton, N.J.: Humana Press, 1990.
26. Cooke I. Paper presented at Recent Advances in Medically Assisted Conception Conference, Geneva, 1991.
27. Jerell J. Personal communication, 1991.
28. Blyth E. Assisted reproduction. What's in it for the children? Children and Society 1990;42:167–182.
29. Raymond C. In vitro fertilization enters stormy adolescence as experts debate the odds. JAMA 1988;259:464–465, 469.
30. Wagner MG, St Clair PA. Are in vitro fertilization and embryo transfer a benefit to all? Lancet 1989;ii:1027–1038.
31. Holme H, Tymstra T. In vitro fertilization in the Netherlands: experiences and opinions of Dutch women. J In Vitro Fertil Embryo Transfer 1987;4:116–123.
32. Williams L. It's going to work for me. Responses to failures of IVF. Birth 1988;15:153–156.
33. Rowe P. Infection and infertility. Geneva: WHO, 1990.
34. Shearer MH. Some effects of assisted reproduction on perinatal care. Birth 1988;15:131–133.
35. Bonnicksen A. Some consumer aspects of in vitro fertilization and embryo transfer. Birth 1988;15:148–152.

PART I

OPTIONS FOR INFERTILE MEN AND WOMEN

1

Medically Assisted Conception:
The State of the Art in Clinical Practice
■

JOSEPH G. SCHENKER

New reproductive technologies proliferate rapidly. Assisted-reproductive technologies in use today include: IVF, GIFT, zygote intrafallopian transfer, pronuclear-stage transfer, tubal intrauterine insemination, fallopian replacement of eggs with delayed intrauterine insemination, and peritoneal oocyte–sperm transfer. IVF and GIFT are the most commonly performed procedures; as such, they are the procedures for which the best data are available. This chapter reviews the indications for IVF and GIFT, the steps involved with each procedure, their clinical results, and factors affecting success rates. The proliferation of IVF programs worldwide. The use of adjunct technologies (embryo cryopreservation, gamete and embryo donation) are also discussed.

INDICATIONS FOR ASSISTED CONCEPTION

In vitro fertilization was developed as a treatment for infertility caused by mechanical tubal factors. The first human IVF pregnancy was achieved in 1976,[1] and the first IVF baby was born in 1978.[2]

During the last 5 years, the indications for IVF have expanded to include male infertility problems, endometriosis, unexplained infertility, and other multiple causes.[3] Some investigators also have used IVF successfully in the treatment of ovulation disorders, anti-sperm antibodies, cervical abnormalities, and genital tract tuber-culosis.[4]

The GIFT technique, first reported by Asch and coworkers in 1984,[5] has achieved wide popularity. The most common indica-tions for this procedure are unexplained infertility, endometriosis, and oligospermia.[6] Candidates must have at least one patent fallo-pian tube that appears anatomically and functionally normal.

Medically assisted conception rarely is indicated as primary treatment for infertility, regardless of the cause. If tubal damage is the underlying cause of infertility, then the options for treatment are microsurgery and assisted-reproductive technologies, especially IVF. The choice will depend on the skills of local clinicians and the extent of tubal damage. Patients who need removal of adhesions or reanastomosis after tubal ligation benefit more from microsurgery: pregnancy rates after microsurgery reach 50% to 80%.[7] However, in cases of severe, postinfectious tubal pathology, the pregnancy rate following surgical treatment is only approximately 15% to 20%.[8] For these cases, IVF may be the first option for treatment.

Tubal surgery is contraindicated in cases of genital tuber-culosis, distal occlusion of tubes with salpingitis isthmica nodosa, and tubes less than 4 cm in length or without fimbria following tubal surgery. In these cases, IVF would be a clear first choice.

In cases of endometriosis, there is indication for medically as-sisted conception if pregnancy does not occur after medical treat-ment using Danazol with or without surgical treatment. However, oocyte recovery rates are much lower in patients with persistent advanced cases of endometriosis.[9]

In cases of male infertility, candidates should be referred for IVF only after failure of other treatment or after prolonged infer-tility. IVF is the final function test for sperm biological activity.

PROCEDURES

At present, stimulation of ovaries with different drug proto-cols to produce multiple follicles and oocytes is standard practice.

No single stimulation protocol, however, can be considered "best." These protocols must be tailored according to individual patient response.

In the future, as methods of embryo culturing and transfer improve, the use of nonstimulated cycles is likely to increase. "Natural-cycle IVF" is an attractive alternative, since it poses fewer risks to the woman and her children. Further, natural-cycle IVF may improve treatment-associated pregnancy rates, because exposure to ovulation-stimulation agents adversely affects the receptivity of the uterine endometrium to implantation.[10]

Oocyte retrieval in humans was first performed in 1966 through laparotomy.[11] A nonsurgical approach was developed in 1972 in which oocytes were flushed from the endometrial cavity,[12] and in 1977, Edwards and Steptoe successfully fertilized human oocytes recovered by laparoscopy.[2]

For some time, laparoscopy was the standard method of oocyte retrieval. However, because of the risks associated with this procedure (complications associated with the use of general anesthesia, damage to viscera and blood vessels, damage to oocytes, and altered pH of follicular fluid from the use of carbon dioxide), it is now used less often.[13, 14] Laparoscopic oocyte retrieval is still used for GIFT, and it also may be combined with diagnostic laparoscopy for infertility investigation.

Ultrasonically guided oocyte collection has become the preferred method for oocyte retrieval. Various techniques exist, including the transabdominal–transvesical approach, the periurethral approach, and the transvaginal approach.[15] Each approach has advantages and disadvantages, but the transvaginal approach is the method of choice in most IVF centers today.[16]

A successful IVF procedure requires the recovery of mature oocytes, with full developmental potential, to undergo normal fertilization and maintain viability throughout cleavage and embryonic development. The maturational stage of the oocytes may vary at the time of their recovery; the assessment of oocyte maturation is performed by morphological criteria before insemination.

The fertilization rates of mature oocytes inseminated with normal sperm are in the area of 17% to 18% in most laboratories.

Fertilization rates are considerably lower, however, when male factors are the underlying cause of infertility.

CLINICAL RESULTS

In 1987, we conducted a worldwide survey of IVF centers. Two hundred and eighty-six centers in the United Kingdom, United States, Australia, New Zealand, France, Asia, Africa, and Israel responded to this survey.[17]

Data are not complete, because not all operating IVF centers participated. It is estimated that the survey covered approximately 40% of the world's activities in assisted conception. More than 30,000 women were treated in these centers in 1987, and 3,913 babies were born following 51,362 treatment cycles and more than 32,000 transfer cycles.

Among the clinics that responded, the average pregnancy rate per 100 treatment cycles was 11.6. Similarly, the pregnancy rate per 100 embryo transfer cycles was 11.5. The live-birth rate per 100 treatment cycles was 7.5.[17]

The rate of spontaneous abortion was 26%. In comparison, the incidence of spontaneous abortions among spontaneous pregnancies commonly is quoted at 10% to 12%.[18] The incidence of extrauterine pregnancy in our data was approximately 5%; among spontaneous conceptions the incidence of extrauterine pregnany is approximately 1%.[19] In addition, approximately 24% of all reported IVF and GIFT pregnancies in our sample were multiple. The expected incidence of multiple pregnancy varies by region, but it generally is in the range of 1% to 2%.[20] These figures are quite comparable to those reported in surveys of IVF programs in Great Britain,[21] Australia and New Zealand,[22] the United States,[23] and France[24] during the same period.

FACTORS AFFECTING SUCCESS RATES

The success of IVF or GIFT procedures very much depends on the underlying cause of infertility. In general, results are best for tubal infertility and worst for infertility caused by male factors.[25]

The age of the women presenting for treatment is another important factor affecting IVF success rates. Pregnancy, and especially live-birth rates, are lower in women over 40 years of age.[26] This may be caused by the higher incidence among older women of spontaneous abortion and pregnancy wastage.[27]

Pregnancy rates are also somewhat affected by ovarian-stimulation protocols. Higher pregnancy rates have been observed in patients when ovulation was induced with gonadotropin-releasing hormone in combination with human menopausal gonadotropin and human chorionic gonadotropin compared with the more traditional combination of human menopausal gonadotropin with clomiphene citrate.[28] As mentioned previously, the choice of stimulation protocols is very much based on individual response; therefore, the mix of patients in any given series comparing stimulation protocols must be taken into account.

Normal embryonic development affects the pregnancy rates resulting from IVF as well. Several factors can affect the quality of an embryo that is fertilized in vitro: the quality of gametes, the timing of insemination, and the culture conditions.[29] At present, we are unable to evaluate correctly an embryo's quality by applying only the parameters of morphological appearance and the rate of cellular division.[30] The optimal stage of development at which to replace a human embryo into the uterus is at the two- to four-cell stage, as practiced by most centers.[31]

A strong relationship exists between the number of embryos transferred and the pregnancy rate. Some centers show a signficant overall linear increase in pregnancy rates that occurs as the number of replaced embryos increases from one to six.[32] However, because the simultaneous transfer of several embryos also greatly increases the chances of multiple pregnancy,[33] many centers limit the number of simultaneously transferred embryos to three.

Both the uterine environment and the quality of the embryo influence implantation. The uterine contribution is difficult to measure, but several factors may have an influence, including pathological changes of the uterine cavity (congenital malformations, myomas, adenomyosis, endometrial tuberculosis, and uterine adhesions), presence of intrauterine infection, and endocrinological factors (synchrony of the development of the embryo with the preparation of uterine endometrium for implantation, endocrine status of the luteal phase, and secretion of uterine proteins required for embryo growth).[34]

GAMETE AND EMBRYO DONATION

Sperm donation is widely practiced, and it has been used for many years in artificial insemination as a treatment for male infertility or in cases where the male partner is the carrier of a serious genetic disease or abnormality. Donor sperm also may be used in assisted-conception programs in cases where treatment with artificial insemination failed after several attempts.[35] In a French study, the pregnancy rate per oocyte retrieval cycle when donor sperm was used was approximately 20% following IVF and 21% following GIFT.[36]

Ovum donation is a new option with several indications: premature menopause; resistant ovary syndrome; autoimmune disorders; galactosemia; and ovarian destruction following surgery, radiation, or hormonal therapy. Oocyte-donation programs face several unresolved problems, however. Oocytes are difficult to freeze and to thaw. Oocyte donors are difficult to obtain, and recipients must receive hormonal replacement therapy to maintain a pregnancy once one is established. The pregnancy rate in ovum donation programs has been reported to be from 25% to 30%.[37,38]

Embryo-donation programs are also underway. The indications for embryo donation include infertility caused by both male and female factors and cases of repeated pregnancy loss.

MICROMANIPULATION OF GAMETES

There have been several reports of pregnancies following injection of spermatozoa under the zona pellucida.[39] Drilling holes or creating slits in the zona pellucida of human oocytes has been used in cases of male infertility.[40, 41]

PROLIFERATION OF ASSISTED CONCEPTION

In 1989, a survey was conducted to estimate the global proliferation of IVF programs. While Australia, New Zealand, the
United Kingdom, Israel, and the Nordic countries have accurate
data on the numbers of IVF clinics, data are incomplete in France,
the United States, and most other countries, making population-
based comparisons of such proliferation unreliable.[42]

Given this limitation we found that as of January 1989, 708
IVF programs existed in 53 countries. Figure 1.1 shows the geographical distribution of these programs. As expected, the majority were located in Western Europe and North America; however,
Oceania had the most IVF programs per unit population, with
North America a close second (Figure 1.2). We also compared the
availability of IVF among countries adjusting for population size
(Figure 1.3), and in these analyses, Israel (with 16 IVF programs
for approximately four million people) by far had the largest number of IVF programs per unit population.

According to our survey, most countries allowed sperm donation. Ovum donation was practiced in at least 17 countries, but
embryo donation was practiced in only 10.

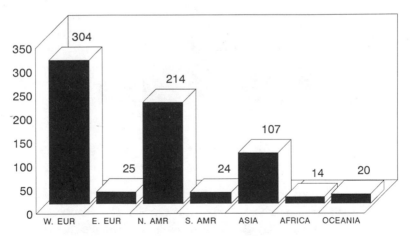

Figure 1.1. Number of IVF units by continent. *(World Survey 1989)*

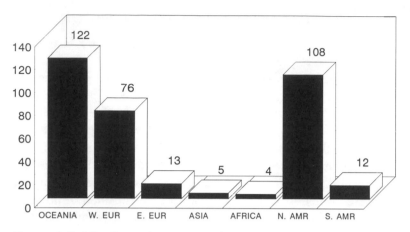

Figure 1.2. Number of IVF units by population. *(World Survey 1989)*

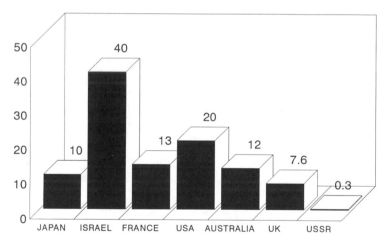

Figure 1.3. Number of IVF units by country. *(World Survey 1989)*

Another international survey of embryo cryopreservation found that 106 IVF centers around the world were freezing embryos as of 31 December 1988.[43] Of the 30,850 embryos frozen, 18,322 survived the freezing–thawing process and 10,290 (56.6%) were judged suitable for replacement; 6,441 replacements occurred, resulting in

632 clinical pregnancies (9.8 pregnancies per 100 embryo-transfer cycles). Three hundred twenty-nine children were born, and 220 pregnancies were still ongoing. The clinical abortion rate was 19%. Four cases of congenital malformations were observed.

CONCLUSIONS

In vitro fertilization, GIFT, and other assisted-reproduction technologies are in widespread use. These technologies are used to treat infertility arising from a number of causes, and they have several associated risks, especially multiple pregnancy, ectopic pregnancy, and spontaneous abortion. Furthermore, the success of treatment as measured by the live-birth rate is modest. Assisted conception, therefore, rarely should be considered as a first option for couples seeking medical treatment for infertility.

REFERENCES

1. Steptoe PC, Edwards RG. Reimplantation of a human embryo with subsequent tubal pregnancy. Lancet 1976;ii:880–881.
2. Steptoe PC, Edwards RG. Birth after reimplantation of a human embryo. Lancet 1978;ii:366.
3. Schenker JG. In vitro fertilization and embryo transfer. Isr J Med Sci 1983;19:218–224.
4. Clark GN. Effect of sperm antibodies in females on human in vitro fertilization. Fertil Steril 1986;46:435.
5. Asch RH, Ellsworth LR, Balmaceda JP, Wong PC. Pregnancy after translaparoscopic gamete intrafallopian transfer. Lancet 1984;iii:1034–1035.
6. The American Fertility Society: Minimal standards for gamete intrafallopian transfer (Gift). Fertil Steril 1988;50:20.
7. Schenker JG, Tanos V. Female sterilization reversal: microsurgery or in vitro fertilization embryo transfer. Presented at the Third International Meeting on Contraception. Heidelburg, Germany, 1990.
8. Winston RML. Additional aspects of tubal surgery: a British perspective. In: Seibel MM, ed. Infertility: A Comprehensive Text. Norwalk: Appleton & Lange, 1990:417–432.
9. Schenker JG. Endometriosis—expert's view. In: Belfort P, ed. Advances

in Gynecology and Obstetrics, Vol. 1. Fertility, Sterility and Contraception. New York: Parthenon, 1989:165–172.

10. Johnston I, Lopata A, Spiers A, et al. In vitro fertilization—the challenge of the eighties. Fertil Steril 1981;36:699.

11. Edwards RG, Donahue RP, Baramki TA, et al. Preliminary attempts to fertilize human oocytes matured in vitro. Am J Obstet Gynecol 1966;96:192–200.

12. Buster JE, Bustillo M, Thorycroft IH, et al. Nonsurgical transfer of in vitro fertilized donated ova to five infertile women: report of two pregnancies (letter). Lancet 1983;ii:223–224.

13. Lenz S, Lauritsen JG. Ultrasonically guided percutaneous aspiration of human follicles under anesthesia. A new method of collecting oocytes for in vitro fertilization. Fertil Steril 1982;38:673–677.

14. Lewin A, Margalioth EJ, Rabinowitz R, et al. Comparative study of ultrasonically guided percutaneous aspiration with local anesthesia and laparoscopic aspiration of follicles in an in vitro fertilization program. Am J Obstet Gynecol 1985;151:621–625.

15. Lewin A, Laufer N, Rabinowitz R, et al. Ultrasonically guided oocyte collection under local anesthesia: the first choice method for in vitro fertilization—a comparative study with laparoscopy. Fertil Steril 1986;46:257–263.

16. Lavy G, Restrepo-Candelo H, Diamond M, et al. Laparoscopic and transvaginal ova recovery: the effect on ova quality. Fertil Steril 1988;49:1002–1006.

17. Schenker JG. Assisted reproduction: formation of ethical laws and regulations. In: Boutaleb Y, Gzouli A, eds. New Conception in Reproduction. New York: Parthenon, 1991:149–155.

18. Hertig AT, Rock J, Adams EC, et al. Thirty-four fertilized human ova, good, bad and indifferent, recovered from 210 women of known fertility: a study of biologic wastage in early human pregnancy. Pediatrics 1959;23:202–211.

19. Schenker JG, Evron S. New concepts in the surgical management of tubal pregnancies and the consequent post-operative results. In: Wallach E, Kempers R, eds. Modern Trends in Infertility and Conception Control. Chicago: Year Book Medical Publishing, 1985:331–351.

20. Schenker JG, Jarkoni S, Granat M. Multiple pregnancies following induction of ovulation. Fertil Steril 1981;35:105–112.

21. Voluntary Licensing Authority for Human In Vitro Fertilization and Embryology: The Fourth Report. London: Royal College of Obstetricians and Gynaecologists, 1989.

22. National Perinatal Statistics Unit, Fertility Society of Australia. IVF and GIFT Pregnancies: Australia and New Zealand 1987. Sydney: University of Sydney, 1988.

23. Medical Research International Society of Assisted Reproductive Technology, the American Fertility Society. In vitro fertilization/embryo transfer in the United States: 1987 results from national IVF-ET registry. Fertil Steril 1989;51:13–19.

24. de Mouzon J, Bellaisch-Allart J, Dubuisson JB, et al. Dossier Fivnat: analyse des resultant 1986. Contracept Fertil Sexual 1987;15:740–746.

25. Acosta A, Kruger T, Swanson RJ, et al. The role of in vitro fertilization in male infertility. Ann N Y Acad Sci 1988;541:297–309.

26. de Mouzon J, Verdasuer S, Cohen J, et al. Dossier Fivnat: analyse de resultant 1988. Contracept Fertil Sexual 1989;17:680–690.

27. Peterson F. The Epidemiology of Early Pregnancy Wastage. Copenhagen: Svenska Bokforlaget Norstedis/Munksgaard, 1966.

28. Gonen Y, Dirnfeld M, Goldman S, et al. The use of long-acting gonadotropin-releasing hormone agonist (GnRH-a; decapeptyl) and gonadotropins versus short-acting GnRH-a (Buseralin) and gonadotropins before and during ovarian stimulation for in vitro fertilization (IVF). J In Vitro Fertil Embryo Transfer 1991;8:254–259.

29. Mohr LR, Trounson AO, Leeton JF, et al. Evaluation of normal and abnormal human embryo development during procedures in vitro. In: Beier HM, Linder HR, eds. Fertilization of the Human Egg In Vitro. Biological Basis and Clinical Application. Berlin: Springer-Verlag, 1983:211–221.

30. Tasarik J. Developmental control of human preimplantation embryos: a comparative approach. J In Vitro Fertil Embryo Transfer 1987;5:347–362.

31. Plachot N. Choosing the right embryo: the challenge of the nineties. J In Vitro Fertil Embryo Transfer 1988;6:100–104.

32. de Mouzon J, Belaisch-Allart J, Cohen J, et al. Dossier Fivnat: analyse des resultants 1987. Contracept Fertil Sexual 1988;16:599–615.

33. Cohen J, Mayaux J, Guihard-Moscato ML. Pregnancy outcome after in vitro fertilization. A collaborative study of 2342 pregnancies. Ann N Y Acad Sci 1988;541:1–6.

34. Lewin A, Laufer N, Yanay N, et al. Double transfer of embryos in in vitro fertilization, or is there a delayed receptivity of the endometrium? J In Vitro Fertil Embryo Transfer 1989;6:139–141.

35. American Fertility Society. New guidelines for the use of sperm donor insemination. Fertil Steril 1986;46(suppl 2).

36. Lansac J, LeLannou D, Imbault M, et al. La grossesse et l'accouchement apres IAD avec sperme congele (Pregnancy following insemination with frozen donor sperm). Rev Fr Gynecol Obstet 1984;79:565–569.

37. Schenker JG. Oocyte and embryo donation. In: Asch RH, ed. Gamete Physiology. Norwell, Mass.: Serono Symposia, 1990:319–329.

38. Schenker JG. Ovum donation: the state of the art. Ann N Y Acad Sci 1988;541:743–754.
39. Ng SS, Bongso A, Ratnam SS, et al. Pregnancy after transfer of sperm under zona. Lancet 1988;ii:790.
40. Schenker JG, Simon A, Laufer N, et al. Micromanipulation of gametes new aspects in assisted reproduction. Harefuah 1989;16:149–151.
41. Gordon JW. Use of micromanipulation for increasing the efficiency of mammalian fertilization in vitro. Ann N Y Acad Aci 1988;541:601–613.
42. Ezra Y, Aceman P, Schenker JG. Update of in vitro fertilization. Isr J Obstet Gynecol 1991;3:149–152.
43. Van Steiteghem AC, Van Abbeel E. World results of human cryopreservation. In: Mashiach S, Ben-Rafael Z, Laufer N, et al., eds. Proceedings of the Sixth World Congress of IVF and Alternate Assisted Reproduction. New York: Plenum Publishers, 1990:601–610.

2

Social Alternatives to Infertility
■

FRANÇOISE LABORIE

THE SOCIAL CONSTRUCTION OF INFERTILITY

Infertility often is described as a tragedy, and this dramatization has been reinforced by the development of the new reproductive technologies. Today the mere presence of a possible medical solution to infertility may increase the pressure on infertile people to make every effort to reproduce.

The dramatization of infertility must be seen within the framework of contemporary social changes. For example, many women are trying to adjust their childbearing to fit their life projects, including career needs. The birth rate has been falling in Europe since 1965 and now is below two children per couple in most European countries. Having fewer children at later ages has increased the value placed on each pregnancy (which must be planned as rationally as possible) as well as on each child born. The recent "pro-birth" and "pro-family" movement in some European countries also adds to this. All these social changes contribute to the perception of infertility as a tragedy.

Despite more liberal views today regarding marriage, cohabitation, and single parenthood, infertility in most countries is seen only as a tragedy for married couples. As Overall noted, "How infertility is evaluated depends upon the total context of the person's life."[1] MacIntyre pointed out that in married women pregnancy and childbearing are normal and desirable, and conversely a desire not to have children is aberrant and in need of explanation, whereas for single women, pregnancy and childbearing are abnormal and undesirable and conversely the desire to have a baby is aberrant, selfish, and in need of explanation. This suggests that infertility is more likely to be perceived as a problem for a married woman than for a single woman.[2]

THE SOCIAL PRODUCTION OF INFERTILITY

The prevalence of infertility is influenced by social behavior. A woman may choose to be sterilized and thereby become infertile; with the aid of IVF, she may revoke this decision and try to become fertile again. Sexually transmitted diseases are a major cause of female and male infertility.[3] Infertility also may be produced iatrogenically.[3]

Until recently, a couple's infertility was assumed to be exclusively female in origin. Often, infertility was the cause of repudiation or divorce, and in many societies this is still the case. It is only recently that male infertility has been discovered and demonstrated in Western societies. Doctors also have begun to talk about the "couple's infertility."

The denial of male sterility can be explained partly by its association with sexual impotence. It is by the female body visibly growing during pregnancy that the man's fertility proves itself. Usually, male infertility is untreatable, but artificial insemination by donor and IVF using donor sperm are palliatives that provide the opportunity for a visible pregnancy that will hide the existence of male infertility (and the impression of impotence) from friends and relations.

Other misconceptions about fertility and infertility are less obvious and are poorly understood. For example, when women gained the freedom to control their fertility through contraception, it was assumed erroneously that when the time came that they wished to have a baby, all they needed to do was to stop using the contraceptive and the desired infant would be immediately conceived. It was not understood that to gain control over not having a baby does not then enable one to gain control over having a baby.

SOCIAL FACTORS AND INFERTILITY

The ability to procreate is far from simply the result of good physiology. Evidence suggests that both psychological and social factors influence the ability to conceive. Some couples seeking infertility treatment have "infertility of unknown origin."[3] In other words, attempts to find a biological cause have failed—the individual appears to function normally biologically yet is infertile. Of course, some infertile people who are classified this way could still have biological causes as yet unknown or undiagnosed; however, it is likely that psychosocial causes may be at the root of the problem for some.

Furthermore, infertile couples who decide to adopt a child frequently will become pregnant soon after this decision is made. One French study showed that among couples with longstanding infertility who then decided to adopt a child, 10% had their own biological child within 2 years of actually beginning the adoption process.[4]

Similarly, infertile couples seeking IVF suddenly may become pregnant before treatment or after the treatment has failed. An Australian study noted that between 1980 and 1985, 450 women registered on the waiting list of a hospital providing IVF wrote to cancel their appointment because they were pregnant.[5] Over a longer period (1980–1988), the same hospital had obtained no more than 275 pregnancies and 138 births after IVF. Thus, there were more treatment-independent pregnancies than pregnancies after treatment with IVF.

Certainly, this observation cannot be taken to mean that treatment-independent pregnancies are psychosocial factors. They simply may be the result of time and continuous trying on the part of the infertile person(s). These observations merely suggest the possibility that at least in some people, proactive decisions may initiate changes in the psychological and social environment, or alter conscious and unconscious processes to the extent that the infertile state is then altered.

INFERTILITY AS A BIOMEDICAL CONSTRUCT

Doctors, as well as the public, tend to seek biological explanations for infertility and solutions through biomedical interventions. Infertility becomes a biomedical construct that leads to profound changes in the way that society views human reproduction. More and more, one finds evidence of the idea that conception can be controlled scientifically and reproduction planned and programmed.

Earlier in history, so-called "blood ties" had been strongly valued in the interest of transmitting name and wealth. Now, with genetics and the new reproductive technologies, these blood ties take on new meaning and social significance as the procreation of one's own DNA. As IVF biologist Jacques Testart pointed out, "Modern genetics has produced the objective supports of genetic egotism and distrust of the stranger, as if the identity of a child could be summed up in the arithmetic of genes: DNA chromosomes are indestructible representations which foster the triumphal narcissism at the hour of procreation."[6]

This renewed genetic imperative reinforces the importance of IVF and related technologies, and it helps to explain the reticence of some infertile people to seek adoption. IVF technology allows the genetic imperative to be fulfilled, at least in part if not in whole. IVF with sperm donation allows the woman's genes to be passed on; IVF with egg donation allows the man's genes to be passed on; and placing a fertilized egg in another woman's uterus allows both the man's and the woman's genes to be passed on.

In France, it is noteworthy that while both IVF with egg donation and IVF with sperm donation are permitted by the National Ethics Committee, embryo donation in which neither the man nor the woman contribute genes is not. Jacques Testart's remark on this is revealing: "This is the new symptom of genetic mystique.

Pure blood is welcomed, half-blood is tolerated, but the stranger is more suspect today than the bastard was yesterday."[6]

In summary, new developments in reproductive technology have an impact on the views of society toward reproduction. The contraceptive advances during the 1960s and 1970s led to the expectation of "have a child if you wish, when you wish." In the 1980s, IVF and the new reproductive technologies led to the expectation of "have your own child, though the price may be high." And the recent combining of IVF with genetic technology may lead to the expectation of "have your child made to order."[7]

SOCIAL ALTERNATIVES
TO MEDICAL MANAGEMENT

Despite the prevailing belief that biomedical technologies are the solution to the problem of infertility, the majority of people who try IVF or a related technology will not become pregnant. There also are many people who, for a variety of reasons, will never seek medical help for their infertility. Therefore, it is important to consider the social alternatives for these infertile people who desire to parent a child.

Adoption

Differences exist among societies in adoption customs, practices, and legislation that depend on their particular social definitions of kinship, family structure, and systems of values and social policies concerning the protection of children. In many societies (especially the African ones), social ties (belonging to a tribe or a clan) are more important than blood ties. The social ties bind the individual to a common ancestor, whether real or mythical. "Children are first children of the clan. They are taken care of by a certain family according to rules of the kinship system and not according to genetic mechanism. Each child is in a certain way the subject of an adoption."[8]

In European countries, adoption has served various functions throughout history. In the countries influenced by Roman law, adoption for a long time remained a device to produce descendants for the purposes of transmission of property, name, and title. It did not, however, exist in the common law, nor in all civil law systems. Officially recorded adoption was very infrequent during the nineteenth century in France. During the twentieth century, adoption has become almost commonplace, resulting from the increased number of orphans after two world wars, the modification of the image of both the abandoned child and the unmarried woman, and the changing patterns of marriage and its functions.

These elements have produced new attitudes. Earlier this century, adoption was viewed with suspicion—adoptive parents were thought to be sterile and adoptive children to be of dubious origin. Today, adoption is considered a unique means of providing parental relationships for children deprived of their natural parents, the normative attitude is that "every child has the right to a family."

In the Western European countries, many more adults are presently seeking adoptive parenthood than there are children available for adoption.[8] France has 20,000 prospective adoptive parents, but the number of wards of the state (adoptable children) has decreased continually, from 100,000 in 1950, 64,000 in 1960, 46,000 in 1970, 22,000 in 1980, 10,400 in 1985, to 7,500 in 1988. Approximately 2,000 to 2,500 new children are placed for adoption each year, but the number of children among them less than 6 months old is very small. Of all adoptable children, 70% are over 12 years old, and 15% suffer from mental or physical handicaps.[8]

Increasingly, prospective adoptive parents have sought children from developing countries that have high birth rates and socioeconomic problems. According to a recent estimate, 15,000 to 20,000 children from developing countries are placed with families in Europe, the United States, Canada and Australia each year.[9] In 1975, 20% to 25% of all adoptions in France involved foreign children. Today, international adoptions represent 50% of all adoptions in France.[8]

Infertility is not the only reason to adopt a child, of course.

Many may wish to adopt for humanitarian reasons. Such people generally do not seek an adoptive child as a substitute for the baby they could not have, and they are likely to adopt children from other countries as well as older and handicapped children.

Some infertile people, however, may consider adoption while continuing medical treatment or only after the medical options have been exhausted. For these prospective adoptive parents, the ideal model of an adoptable child generally is that of a young, healthy, white baby. Having gone through the process of mourning the loss of procreation, they would at least like to live an experience comparable to other parents (i.e., to care for a newborn infant). However, regarding their actual experiences, people who have gone through IVF and later adopted a child point out that with IVF, the focus is on the needs of the adults involved, but with adoption, the focus shifts to the needs of the child. For this reason, they experience adoption as a less egotistical process than IVF. Thus, if infertile people are able to overcome the new genetic imperative mentioned previously, then adoption is seen by them as an acceptable alternative.

Many people have reservations before adopting. Some are afraid of the inquisitorial procedures necessary before they can be approved as adoptive parents. Many feel impatient with the long waiting period, and some express concern that the children may have psychological scars from earlier experiences or eventually will search for their "biological" parents.

Despite such reservations, parents usually speak in a very different manner once the child has been adopted. They discover certain advantages to adoption of which they were previously unaware. For a couple with infertility, adoption has the advantage of putting the two members of the couple (the one who is infertile and the one who is not) on equal footing concerning their relations to child; in other words, unlike when one parent is genetically linked to the child, neither parent is kinship-tied with an adopted child.

Parents who adopt and are infertile often emphasize the opportunities that adoption has brought to them, for example, the extraordinary experience of having to educate a child from an-other culture or a handicapped child. In addition, some state that despite their infertility, adoption has served to prove the "fertility" (i.e., the strength and stability) of the couple. A description of one person's experience is illustrative:

> Living continually with regrets or with a permanent hope of possible pregnancy, that is for me "genuine sterility", because this hope is often paralysing. But I think that being able to forget the past and turn towards the future may be infinitely more difficult for couples who don't know why "it's not working". What remains today of our problem of sterility? The memory of an ordeal, but who does not have any? Isn't losing a child a thousand times worse? Depending upon the respective personalities of the partners and the manner in which they support each other, a couple's sterility can be a factor for rupture, for sclerosis, for gazing at one's navel. However it can also be a step towards a profound knowledge and under-standing of each other, a formidable cement of the couple. And once the worst part of the disappointment—legitimate disappointment—is passed by, most of us are able to continue on with a perfectly satisfactory sex life without constraint.[10]

Speaking about the period where this person had recourse to med-ical treatment, she adds:

> I was obstinate to the point of undergoing two trips to the operating room; I have had two extra-uterine pregnancies with rupture of the tubes. The first which was not diagnosed in time really put my life in danger. Physically, I took a year to put myself back together again. Psychologically, the first post-operative months were very hard. I was at the end of my tether, in spite of my husband's love. I kept on trying to find biological solutions, and I read everything which was pub-lished on the first IVF attempts in Great Britain. Finally, I renounced definitely without regret: it was too risky for the child to be born and very problematic to foresee such manipu-lations. But on the other hand, to the surprise of many, I expe-rienced for several months a very real wounding of my ego, something which now makes me smile. For I was capable of brilliantly succeeding in many things that are difficult for many people, notably my university exams, and here I was

completely inept at doing what everybody can do without having learnt. It is provoking, isn't it?[10]

And finally:

> Thus we turned to adoption. Certain people will think we could have—thus should have—taken this step earlier. They think we would have gained time, given the long waiting time. I am sure of the contrary. Launching on the adoption procedure, one needs to give all of oneself to have a chance of arriving. It is thus necessary to be resolutely turned towards the future without any tears in one's eyes, being back in form, setting up a well-joined and balanced couple. The child can be "himself": no question of dreaming that he will embody the qualities the child we could have made, would have had. . . . Just have to try to put yourself in the shoes of those responsible for adoption! Would you take the risk of committing a child to the care of a couple whose thoughts are only turned towards continuing to get treatments in order to make their "own" child? Or to an undecided couple still too close to the regret of not having had their child?[10]

Regarding the legislative and judicial policies, considerable differences exist among countries in laws concerning adoption. These differences concern:

1. The way in which adoption is performed (by private contract, the state acting only to authorize the agreement; or by judicial decree)
2. The conditions for adoption, including age and age differences between adopter and adoptee, civil status of adoptive parents, and presence of other children as an impediment to adoption
3. Its legal effects, including the establishment of a legal relationship with the relatives of the adopters, the acquisition of citizenship, and succession rights
4. The conditions of revocation

Over the past two or three decades, however, the trend in most countries is toward giving the greatest weight to the interests of the child and integrating the child into the adopting family, severing all legal bonds with the natural family, informing children not only of the fact that they have been adopted but also of their family background. Furthermore, the conditions for adoption tend to become less strict to facilitate adoptions, for example, the presence of previous legitimate children as an impediment to the adoption of children is disappearing. In those countries that restrict adoption to children, the trend is toward lowering the maximum age (for example, 15 years in France and 14 years in Spain and Portugal). Adoption now generally entails complete assimilation of the adopted child into the adopting family. The requirement of a trial period, fixed by law or determined by court in each individual case, is commonplace, and a trend toward reducing the possibilities of revoking adoption also exists. Finally, in many countries, governments have become more involved not only with adoption but also with foster placement of children.

Concerning international law for private, intercountry adoption, there is a clear trend toward giving paramount consideration to the best interests of the child. In Europe, there is a tendency for the law of the adopters' country and not that of the prospective adoptive child to govern most of the questions concerning the conditions of the adoption (particularly questions of consent).

Voluntary childlessness

There seems to be a consensus that the number of people choosing to remain childless is increasing, at least in those industrialized countries where numbers of women working outside the home, levels of education, divorce rates, and standards of living are increasing. People choosing to remain childless receive mixed messages from society, which on the one hand insists on the importance of preserving the genetic make-up of the group (and views voluntary childlessness as "selfish") and, on the other, supports family planning because of the global population crisis (and views voluntary childlessness as "selfless").

Voluntary childlessness generally is regarded as the prerogative of fertile people. However, a proportion of people do opt for childlessness on learning they are infertile. They may or may not have their infertility medically confirmed, but in any case, they never present for treatment of infertility. Others may try medical treatment for a time, then choose to drop out and be satisfied with childlessness. Finally, there is the most visible group; those who choose this option only after all medical options have failed.

That part of the medical community promoting IVF has, of course, only come in contact with this latter group; therefore, they have a distorted perception of the wishes of infertile people. Clinicians and social scientists alike, who only interact with this highly self-selected group, have developed an image of the infertile woman as desperate and willing to undergo any treatment, no matter what the risks, no matter what the cost, to achieve motherhood. These also are the people who have organized into pressure groups to promote government funding of IVF services. The infertile choosing voluntary childlessness, adoption, or other social options initially have not participated in the politics of the new reproductive technologies.

Because of all the mixed messages and confusion over voluntary childlessness, it is important to gain more information on this option. At the same time, this option needs to be presented to infertile people, along with the other options, when they ask for advice.

Voluntary waiting

Choosing to wait for a time before making a decision regarding treatment of infertility can be a positive step. As so many people on waiting lists for adoption or IVF have found, waiting often results in a spontaneous natural pregnancy. Making a definite decision to wait and "take a break" removes the pressures and may allow an opportunity for healing from the traumas that treatments such as IVF so often entail. Ironically, the sex life of someone undergoing treatment of infertility may be seriously disturbed, with loss of spontaneity and intimacy.

While some clinicians label a couple as infertile after only a few months of attempting to become pregnant, others recognize the value of waiting—or at least the avoidance of overly enthusiastic use of aggressive treatment. As one French gynecologist wrote, "Recommending to women to do nothing is a possible therapeutic attitude, too often neglected."[11] Through waiting, the best option to pursue often becomes clear.

CONCLUSIONS

Infertile people, policy makers, and the public at large are caught between two very different views of infertility: the biomedical construct that defines infertility as a disease needing medical treatment, and the social construct that defines it as a social problem dealt with in any number of ways depending on the needs, wishes, and preferences of the infertile couple and the resources available in the community. Because a strong leaning toward the biomedical construct exists, little or no attempt has been made to design services that bring together all options for infertile people. Infertile people are left to muddle through as best they can, learning the hard way the true costs and benefits of each option explored. Similarly, there has been no attempt on the part of policy makers to bridge the gap between the social care system (adoption and foster care services) and the medical system (new and not-so-new reproductive technologies). Policy makers discuss at length IVF and the relative merits of including it as a health service in national health insurance schemes, but rarely do they discuss the problem of infertility in the community and what to do about it.

No one knows how many infertile people choose social or medical solutions. Very little is known about the attitudes and preferences of infertile people to various solutions, or about how their attitudes and preferences change as a result of exposure to various options. It is likely that attitudes and preferences will differ from country to country and even among subpopulations within a given country. Research on attitudes and preferences of infertile people toward social and medical options is needed for the rational planning of infertility services.

Given the separateness of the social and medical systems in

nearly every country (each system has its own practitioners, regulations, funding mechanisms, and so forth), and given that this situation is not likely to change, what can be done to help infertile people navigate their way through the various options available? One quite successful strategy has been tried by certain feminist centers in Frankfurt and Berlin: the formation of self-help and counseling groups for infertile women. These groups were formed to give women an opportunity to clarify the motives behind their desire for children without attempting to either validate or negate these feelings. The groups also provide information about all options—social and medical—so that women can decide their own best course of action (or inaction) to pursue. The groups are not supported by any special interest group or attached to any service, so there is no built-in bias toward one solution or another. Furthermore, the self-help approach allows women to come into contact with and seek support from other women experiencing the same problem. The formation of such groups in other countries would be a low-cost, potentially effective means of providing both information and assistance to infertile women (and men) to enable and empower them to make informed and rational choices.

Beyond this rather practical approach, there also is a need for more information on the contribution of the various solutions in a given society, services to assist the infertile in considering all options, and laws and regulations that allow choice and greater access of infertile people to all options with approximately equal cost and waiting time. These are the challenges for governments and their policy makers.

REFERENCES

1. Overall C. Ethics and Human Reproduction. A Feminist Analysis. Boston: Allen & Unwin, 1987:141.
2. MacIntyre S. Who wants babies? The social construction of "instincts." In: Leonard Baker D, Allen S, eds. Sexual Divisions and Society: Process and Change. London: Tavistock, 1976:159.
3. U.S. Congress Office of Technology Assessment. Infertility: Medical

and Social Choices. Washington D.C.: U.S. Government Printing Office, 1988.

4. Progress. Newsletter of the Special Programme of Research, Development and Research Training in Human Reproduction. Geneva: WHO, World Bank, UNDP, UNFPA no. 15, 1990.

5. Saunders DM, Matthews M, Lancaster PAL. The Australian Register: current research and future role. Ann N Y Acad Sci 1988;541:7–21.

6. Testart J. Don adoption des oeufs humains. Autrement. Abandon et Adoption 1988;96:185.

7. Spallone P, Steinberg DL, eds. Made to Order: The Myth of Reproductive and Genetic Progress. Oxford: Pergamon Press, 1987.

8. Comillon M, Duyme M. Indication sociologiques et historiques sur l'adoption. In: L'adoption une Famille pour un Enfant. Paris: Institut de l'Enfance et de la Famille, 1988.

9. Note on the desirability of preparing a new convention on international cooperation in respect to intercountry adoption, drawn up by Hans Van Loon, December 1987, for the Permanent Bureau of the Hague Conference (6, Scheveningseweg 2517 KT the Hague, the Netherlands).

10. Vivre la sterilité. Accueil 1983;6:13–15.

11. Cabau A. Pour que l'enfant paraisse. Comprendre et combattre l'infertilite. Paris: Ed Flammarion, 1990.

PART II

TECHNOLOGY ASSESSMENT

3

Technology Assessment and Infertility Care

■

H. DAVID BANTA

> *If the Lord Almighty had consulted me before embarking upon the Creation, I would have recommended something simpler.*
> —ALFONSO X OF CASTILE

Our time is full of challenges and opportunities, and observers often echo the bewilderment of Alfonso X: it is just too complex to deal with. Among the many challenges, that posed by rapid technological change is one of the most pressing.

Technological change in health care is not a situation to decry. Much of the present-day health care technology is inefficient or only marginally effective. Much of it is empirical and never has been adequately assessed. The future will witness the replacement of most technology presently in use.

How will decisions about replacement be made? Will it be in response to the claims of medical specialists? In response to the economic needs of industry? In response to concerns about increasing health care budgets and expenditures? Or is it possible to base these replacement decisions on valid information using a strategic approach to the assessment of health care technology?

THE NEED FOR TECHNOLOGY ASSESSMENT

During its development, a given technology must pass through a stage of being considered "experimental." Unfortunately, the transition from "experimental" to "accepted" technology all too often has little to do with rational assessment. In practice, "accepted" tends to mean accepted by the medical profession.

Perhaps the most classic example is that of gastric freezing.[1] During the mid-1950s, a surgeon developed a device to treat peptic ulcer disease by circulating very cold alcohol through the stomach for the purpose of freezing the stomach to kill acid-producing cells. In 1962, he reported no serious side effects, reduced stomach acid output, and radiographical evidence of ulcer healing. By the end of 1963, 1,000 of these devices had been sold in the United States, and 15,000 procedures using the device had been performed. Subsequently, reports of patient harm—and even death—resulting from treatment with the device appeared. The device fell rapidly out of use, and clinical trials published in 1964 showed no benefit. By 1966, the technique was rarely used.

The case of diethystilbestrol (DES) also illustrates how an improper evaluation of benefits and safety can lead to iatrogenesis. Diethystilbestrol was introduced during the late 1930s and, based on a number of badly designed studies, was promoted as a treatment for pregnancy complications.[2] Controlled studies in the 1950s showed no benefit from treatment with the drug[3] but widespread use continued throughout the world. In 1970, however, a rare type of vaginal cancer was discovered in young women whose mothers had taken DES during pregnancy.[4] Since then, a number of other complications have become evident in both the sons and daughters of these mothers. The drug gradually fell out of use during the 1970s.

Such cases showed policy makers and the public that medical opinion regarding the benefits and risks of a health technology was not sufficient evidence to justify its widespread clinical application. It became clear that a system for assessing technology was needed to provide valid information for rational planning.

THE PHILOSOPHY OF TECHNOLOGY ASSESSMENT

The main purpose of health care technology assessment is to help ensure that health care technologies are efficacious (or effective), safe, and are used appropriately. Efficacy is the probability that a particular medical technology, under ideal conditions of use, will benefit people in a defined population who have a specific medical problem. Effectiveness is similar, except that it refers to the usual conditions of use. Safety is a judgment of the acceptability of the risks involved in treatment. Risk is expressed as the probability of harm to people in a defined population associated with the use of a medical technology applied for a specific medical problem under specified conditions of use.[5]

The most important method for testing both the efficacy and safety of a medical technology is the randomized clinical trial. This allows one to compare therapeutic and untoward outcomes in patients treated with a new technology, placebo, or another form of therapy. Random assignment of patients to treatment conditions is a method of controlling for extraneous factors (both known and unknown) that may be associated with outcome.

Other methods for assessing safety include follow-up and case-control studies. Follow-up studies of patients treatment with a technology maybe carried out to examine associations between exposure to the treatment and rare, untoward effects. Case-control studies match a group of people with a specific disease or condition to a similar group without the condition. Factors present in those with the disease but absent in the control group may explain the difference.

It often is not enough to know that a health care technology is beneficial and safe when used appropriately. One also must establish that the benefit to be gained is worth the cost incurred. Policy makers must allocate money and other resources in a way that will maximize the health and well-being of the population. Resources allocated to particular health problems might be better applied to other health problems or even to other areas of societal activity if they achieve a greater impact on health and well-being.

Cost-effectiveness and cost–benefit analyses are the techniques used to compare the negative and positive consequences of alternative programs or technologies. Briefly, the difference between cost–benefit and cost-effectiveness analyses is this: in cost–benefit analysis, all consequences are valued in monetary terms; the cost-effectiveness analysis, desirable consequences of a program or technology are valued in some other way. Because of the difficulty in assigning a monetary value to various states of health, cost–benefit analysis has serious limitations. Cost-effectiveness analysis, however, permits comparison of the costs per unit of effectiveness among competing, alternative programs or technologies.[6]

As a formal evaluation technique, cost-effectiveness analysis is used to assess decisions concerning resource allocation. This analysis can be very helpful to decision makers, because the technique can lend structure to the problem under study, allow consideration of the key effects of a decision, and force the statement of key assumptions.

Cost-effectiveness analysis is a useful aid in decision-making, but it does have weaknesses. Both costs and benefits are difficult to predict precisely, and intangible benefits are difficult to value. Also, considerations of equity, culture, and politics must be incorporated as well.

Furthermore, the social consequences and ethical questions imposed by a technology must be considered in all decisions concerning health care, and this evaluation must be considered a legitimate part of assessing technology.[7] In its broadest form, a technology assessment would consider all aspects of the technology, including its "second-order" impacts. Such a comprehensive assessment rarely is done in the health field, perhaps because efficacy and cost-effectiveness (or the lack thereof) usually seem to be more pressing issues. In the case of IVF, however, a broader view is essential.

"Appropriate use" also must be seen in a cultural context. Western society has become increasingly technological, and what is seen as appropriate in Europe differs from what is appropriate in Asia or Africa. Great differences in the diffusion and use of technology also are seen when comparing individual European countries. Therefore, the cultural and social dimensions need to be considered more often in technology assessments.

A complete system for technology assessment would require monitoring of the entire universe of health care technology (both existing and new), evaluating each technology at various points in its life cycle, and conducting multiple evaluations to ensure correct results and coverage of all potentially important effects. The information from this assessment would be summarized and furnished to policy makers, health care providers, and the public. Needless to say, this model seldom is followed; in practice, important decisions are driven not by rational planning but by the power relationships within a society.

IN VITRO FERTILIZATION

In the case of IVF, decision-making has been distressingly ad hoc. IVF technology has been allowed to proliferate rapidly, and this proliferation appears to have no relation to an assessment of its role in infertility care. For example, in the Netherlands, IVF has been seen as a potential policy issue since the birth of the first IVF baby in 1978. The government asked for advice on IVF in 1983, and in 1984, the Dutch Health Council recommended that the number of IVF centers be limited to only the eight academic hospitals.[8] The government announced it would limit the number of centers by its powers under Article 18 of the Hospital Provisions Act, but then did not act. The results of a cost-effectiveness analysis indicated that five centers would be an efficient number,[9] but 12 programs developed nonetheless, with 30 or more clinical centers associated with them. Finally, in February 1990, the government announced that it would grant licenses to all 12 IVF programs.

The Netherlands is not alone. In France, IVF and related technologies have been allowed to proliferate unchecked, and the number of programs currently in operation is estimated to be approximately 150. This is well over twice the number of programs licensed by the government, but as yet, no action has been taken to enforce practice regulations or to close the unlicensed centers.

Similar struggles over regulation and control of technology are occurring in the United Kingdom, Germany, Australia, and Israel. The point is that technology assessment itself cannot be of much value in the absense of clear health policy decisions, regulatory control, and enforcement.[10]

THE ROLE OF INDUSTRY

Industry is the largest supporter of medical research and the assessment of health care technology. It also is the most important source of information on new health care technology. Industry's role in technology assessment is crucial, because it would be impossible to replace this support with public funds. The information it produces, however, is aimed at promoting new drugs and devices and not optimizing medical practice or health.

Industry is a driving force behind the proliferation of IVF programs. Because drugs and devices are used, IVF is a potentially profit-making enterprise. In the Netherlands, industry supported the travel of Dutch physicians to established IVF centers for training, and it sponsored national conferences to promote the advancement of this technology. Industry also continues to support certain Dutch IVF programs with funds for both research and travel.

MEDICAL ALTERNATIVES:
SOME PROMISING EXAMPLES

While IVF has been proliferating, alternative medical treatments have been developed that in time may replace it as the treatment of choice for infertility. For example, microsurgery or laser treatment using the laparoscope may be superior options for women with occluded fallopian tubes, a frequent cause of infertility. Pregnancy rates following surgical repair of the fallopian tubes have increased greatly since the introduction of microsurgery, and the most successful series report continuing pregnancy rates of 25% to 30%.[11]

In a limited number of publications, results of fertility-promoting procedures with the carbon-dioxide laser have been discussed. Tulandi[12,13] and Tulandi and colleagues[14,15] published several randomized, clinical trials comparing laser laparoscopy of tubal infertility with microsurgical procedures. Pregnancy rates were comparable in all studies, and they varied between 21% and 41% with these two procedures.

Endometriosis is another fairly common cause of infertility, and danazol is the standard treatment. A new treatment using a laser applied through a laparoscope, either alone or in conjunction with danazol, appears to be successful; ongoing pregnancy rates between 30% and 70% have been reported.[16-21]

In contrast, each IVF procedure has a success rate of approximately 10%. IVF does not cure infertility, and the procedure must be repeated each time a pregnancy is desired. If a woman becomes pregnant once after treatment with laser or microsurgery, however, she can become pregnant again without undergoing another course of treatment.

THE PLACE OF IN VITRO FERTILIZATION IN INFERTILITY SERVICES

Why has IVF become the accepted treatment for infertility, displacing other medical technologies that could be more effective? Perhaps it is a matter of excitement, the image of technological sophistication, or a medical "fad." No doubt a place exists for IVF in infertility services, but in time, it may prove to be the alternative of last resort. Newer techniques may prove to be safer, more effective, and provide a cure for infertility and not just a one-time opportunity for pregnancy. It is important that these new techniques be evaluated properly in clinical trials where they can be compared with no treatment and treatment with IVF.

Today, the situation regarding medically assisted conception and the new reproductive technologies is profoundly irrational. The field cries out for medical decision analysis and definition of appropriate therapeutic processes. Application of the principles and methods of technology assessment has enormous potential to improve infertility care, and it also can help assure that resources are well spent. This will become more crucial as decision makers struggle to determine the value of technologies within health care systems.

REFERENCES

1. Fineberg HV. Gastric freezing: a study of diffusion of medical innovation. In: Committee on Technology in Health Care. Medical Technology and the Health Care System. Washington, D.C.: National Academy of Sciences, 1979:173–200.
2. Apfel RJ, Fisher SM. To Do No Harm: DES and the Dilemmas of Modern Medicine. London: Yale University Press, 1984.
3. Dieckmann WJ, Davies ME, Ryunkiewicz LM, Pottinger RE. Does the administration of diethystilbestrol during pregnancy have therapeutic value? Am J Obstet Gynecol 1953;66:1062–1081.
4. Herbst AL, Poskanzer DC, Robboy SJ, et al. Prenatal exposure to stilbestrol: a prospective comparison of exposed female offspring with unexposed controls. N Engl J Med 1975;292:334–339.
5. Office of Technology Assessment. Assessing the Efficacy and Safety of Medical Technologies. Washington, D.C.: U.S. Government Printing Office, 1982.
6. Office of Technology Assessment. Implications of cost-effectiveness analysis of medical technology. Washington, D.C.: U.S. Government Printing Office, 1982.
7. Banta HD, Behney CJ, Willems JS. Toward a Rational Technology in Medicine. New York: Springer, 1981.
8. Gezondheidraad. Interimadvies Inzake In Vitro Fertilisatie. Den Haag: Gezondheidsraad, 1984.
9. Haan G. Effecten en Kosten Van In Vitro Fertilisatie, een Prospektieve Multicener Studie. Dissertation. Maastricht: University of Limburg, 1989.
10. de Wit A, Banta HD. The diffusion of in vitro fertilization in the Netherlands and England. Int J Technol Assess Health Care 1991; 7:574–584.
11. Soules MR. Infertility surgery. In: DeCherney AH, ed. Reproductive Failure. New York: Churchill Livingstone, 1986.

12. Tulandi T. Reconstructive tubal surgery by laparoscopy. Obstet Gynecol Surv 1987;42:193–198.
13. Tulandi T. Salpingo-ovariolysis: a comparison between laser surgery and electrosurgery. Fertil Steril 1986;45:489–491.
14. Tulandi T, Vilos GA. A comparison between laser surgery and electrosurgery for bilateral hydrosalpinx: a two-year follow-up. Fertil Steril 1985;44:846–848.
15. Tulandi T, Sirag R, McInnes RA, et al. Reconstructive surgery of hydrosalpinx with and without the carbon dioxide laser. Fertil Steril 1984;42:839–842.
16. Chong AP. Danazol vs carbon dioxide laser plus postoperative danazol: treatment of infertility due to mild pelvic endometriosis. Lasers Surg Med 1985;5:571–576.
17. Chong AP. Infertility amenable to laser surgery. In: Baggish MS, ed. Basic and Advanced Laser Surgery in Gynecology. Norwalk: Appleton-Century-Crofts, 1985.
18. Chong AP, Baggish MS. Management of pelvic endometriosis by means of intraabdominal carbon dioxide laser. Fertil Steril 1984; 41:14–19.
19. Kelly RW, Roberts DK. CO_2 laser laparoscopy. A potential alternative to danazol in the treatment of stage I and II endometriosis. J Reprod Med 1983;28:638 640.
20. Keye WR. The present and future application of lasers to the treatment of endometriosis and infertility. Int J Fertil 1986;31:160–164.
21. Nezhat C, Crowgey S, Nezhat F. Videolaparoscopy for the treatment of endometriosis associated with infertility. Fertil Steril 1989;51:237–240.

4

The Effectiveness of In Vitro Fertilization:
An Epidemiological Perspective
■

FIONA J. STANLEY *and* SANDRA M. WEBB

This chapter discusses the effectiveness of IVF and related technologies such as GIFT. (Any general reference to IVF in this chapter includes related procedures such as GIFT.) Topics include the current data on effectiveness, problems of definition, data collection and reporting, deficiencies in the classification of infertility, and inconsistencies in evaluating the outcomes of therapy. Also, suggestions are made on how to assess properly the effectiveness of IVF treatment and what types of data should be collected for ongoing monitoring of IVF services.

EFFECTIVENESS

In clinical parlance, IVF effectiveness rates are referred to as "success rates." Success rates can appear either optimistic or dismal depending on the numerators and denominators used in their calculation. For this reason, the numerator and denominator of a success rate must be defined precisely.

In vitro fertilization consists of a series of treatment phases. A woman may drop out of treatment at any phase because the treatment failed; therefore, when calculating success rates, using em-

Table 4.1.
EFFICACY IN IVF BY CHOICE OF NUMERATOR
AND DENOMINATOR

NUMERATOR/DENOM-INATOR	EFFICACY, %		
	United Kingdom, 1987	*United States, 1987*	*Australia, 1988*
Egg collections/treatment cycles	78.5	74.0	86.3
Embryo transfers/treatment cycles	62.8	64.1	72.3
Pregnancies/treatment cycles	11.0	11.6	11.6
Live births/treatment cycles	8.5	8.4	8.1
Clinical pregnancies/embryo transfers	17.5	18.1	16.0
Live births/embryo transfers	13.6	13.1	11.2
Spontaneous abortions/treatment cycles	2.3	2.9	2.6
Ectopic pregnancies/treatment cycles	0.7	0.9	0.8
Perinatal death/treatment cycles	0.4	—	—
Spontaneous abortion/clinical pregnancies*	20.9	25.2	22.1
Ectopic pregnancies/clinical pregnancies*	6.6	7.5	6.6
Perinatal death/clinical pregnancies*	3.3	—	4.2
Live births/clinical pregnancies*	77.6	72.5	69.8

*The definitions of pregnancy are inconsistent between countries. For example, the term excludes ectopic pregnancy in the U.S. data, while this is included in the Australian data. For the U.K. data, the term is unclear.

bryo-transfer cycles as the denominator will increase the rate while using all started treatments will decrease the rate. Similarly, if clinical pregnancies are used as the measure of success then spontaneous abortion and, depending on the definition of clinical pregnancy used, ectopic pregnancy, stillbirth, and preterm birth are all counted as successes of treatment; in this case the rate is inflated. If live birth (and especially live birth at term) is the outcome of interest, then success rates are modest. Table 4.1 illustrates the variation in effectiveness depending on the choice of both numerator and denominator.

CORRELATES OF SUCCESS

The success of IVF is not the same for everyone. IVF effectiveness is determined in large measure by client characteristics, clinic characteristics, and variations in the application of the procedures themselves.

Regarding client characteristics, success rates vary depending on the underlying cause of infertility. For example, women treated because of either male factors or severe endometriosis are much less likely to benefit from IVF compared with women having bilateral tubal blockage and functioning ovaries.[1-3] Success rates also diminish for older women and for women who have remained infertile for longer periods of time.[3]

Success rates vary markedly among clinics as well. Clinic success rates depend on the experience of the physicians and the staff, the mix of clients they serve, and the size (treatment capacity) of the clinic itself.[4-6] Clinics that admit for treatment more difficult cases naturally will meet with less success, and inexperienced clinicians or clinicians working in clinics delivering fewer than 100 treatment cycles per year generally have below-average success rates (Tables 4.2 and 4.3).

Regarding the procedures themselves, much available data, such as from the U.K. registry, show the number of eggs or embryos transferred during IVF or GIFT has a major bearing on success rates (Table 4.4). For this reason, multiple egg and embryo

Table 4.2.

RELATIONSHIP BETWEEN IVF TREATMENTS PER YEAR AND LIVE BIRTHS AFTER IVF AND EMBRYO TRANSFER

IVF CYCLES PER YEAR, *n*	UNITED STATES, 1987			UNITED KINGDOM, 1987			AUSTRALIA, 1988		
	Clinics, n	Total transfers, n	Live births per transfer, %	Clinics, n	Total transfers, n	Live births per transfer, %	Clinics, n	Total transfers, n	Live births per transfer, %
< 100	73	2474	11.1	14	249	5.2	6	175	11.4
> 100	23	5087	14.1	20	5343	14.0	18	6470	11.1

Table 4.3.

RELATIONSHIP BETWEEN GIFT TREATMENTS PER YEAR AND LIVE BIRTHS AFTER TREATMENT*

GIFT CYCLES PER YEAR, *n*	UNITED STATES, 1987			AUSTRALIA, 1988		
	Clinics, n	Total transfers, n	Live births per transfer, %	Clinics, n	Total transfers, n	Live births per transfer, %
< 100	63	720	13.5	14	449	15.4
> 100	8	1248	21.2	10	2173	21.1

*U.K. data unavailable.

Table 4.4.
PREGNANCY RATES PER EMBRYO/GIFT
TRANSFER IN THE UNITED KINGDOM, 1987

	PREGNANCY, %	
EGGS OR EMBRYOS TRANSFERRED, *n*	IVF	GIFT
1	6.5	1.7
2	11.8	10.4
3	21.0	18.6
4	21.9	18.9
5 or more	3.9	37.2

transfer is common, even though it places women at risk for multiple pregnancy.[7] The American Fertility Society found that in 66.2% of embryo-transfer cycles recorded in their data base, three or more (up to a total of nine) embryos were transferred.[6] Also, the Australia/New Zealand IVF register noted an increase over time in the number of IVF cycles in which at least three embryos were transferred, from 46.6% in 1979–1983 to 78.4% in 1987.[4] However, in 1988 Australian practitioners recommended that the number of embryos transferred should not exceed three. In the United Kingdom the code of practice under the Human Fertilisation and Embryology Act now places a similar restriction.

RANDOMIZED CLINICAL TRIALS

Presently, the best available data on IVF effectiveness come from IVF registries. These registries pool data from all or some fraction of clinics performing IVF within a given country or region, but these data do not reveal the true success of IVF. To determine its true effectiveness, IVF must be compared with other treatments for infertility and with no treatment at all.

The best method to estimate the effectiveness (efficacy) of a medical treatment is the randomized clinical trial. Such a trial randomly allocates patients to treatment and no-treatment (and sometimes alternative treatment) groups. Without this experimental study design, information on the effectiveness (and risks) of treatment is limited by selection bias, selective losses to follow-up, and failure to control for extraneous or confounding variables.

Despite the increasing number of published therapeutic trials for infertility treatments, by 1989, only 8.6% of 70 clinical trials of infertility treatment excluding IVF were of a randomized, controlled design.[8] In many of these studies, the methodology employed was so flawed as to render their results and conclusions meaningless. To date, there has been no published randomized clinical trial that fully evaluates IVF effectiveness, but at least one has been completed as part of the Canadian Royal Commission into the New Reproductive Technologies.

Randomized clinical trials may prove that IVF has limited value, at least for many individuals. Several studies show that 7% to 28% of couples accepted for IVF programs conceive spontaneously, either while on the waiting list or within 2 years of treatment.[7] Using statistical modeling for a group of couples unable to conceive for 3 years, Leridon and Spira[9] estimated that the proportion achieving a pregnancy in the fourth year could be as high as 48%. Although considerable problems arise from the lack of comparability between these studies, the message is clear: a proportion of women accepted into IVF programs subsequently will achieve a pregnancy without treatment. It is of the utmost importance, therefore, to determine by means of randomized clinical trials whether IVF is more beneficial than alternative medical treatment or no treatment at all for varying causes and durations of infertility. The design and conduct of these trials would, however, present considerable methodological, practical, and ethical difficulties.

LIFE TABLES FOR COMPARISONS OF INFERTILITY MANAGEMENT

The use of life-table methods in the analysis of infertility treatments was recommended strongly by Cramer and colleagues,[10] and most would agree that life tables have considerable advantages over crude pregnancy rates. Olive[11] also supports this method as well as other sequential methods, particularly for use with randomized clinical trials. Calculating accumulating likelihood of pregnancy from fecundability as presented by Jansen[12] also is an acceptable method for comparison. (Fecundability is a couple's monthly probability of conceiving calculated from empirical data.)

The first requirement for a life table is a well-defined starting point for each patient. This could vary depending on the method of intervention used, but it should be defined for each study and before randomization occurs in a trial. It must be applied uniformly in all those trials whose data are included in the life table.

The second requirement is a well-defined end point. As the end point determines exit from one column of the table, it only can be dichotomous (yes or no) and must occur only once for each subject. (Each new cycle can begin as a new subject in the life table.) These end points can be chosen by referring to the list of numerators and denominators presented earlier.

The value of a life-table analysis is that it corrects for varying lengths of follow-up and for the losses to follow-up. If the sample size is large enough, then the variance for each data point is small and the life table becomes a smooth curve.

DATA FOR ONGOING MONITORING

In response to calls for better data on IVF effectiveness, in several countries IVF registries for the ongoing collection and reporting of data related to treatment effectiveness and risks have been organized through legislation or professional societies. As previously mentioned, such pooled data does not provide complete information on the effectiveness of treatment; however, at least in the foreseeable future, it is the best available source of data regarding this. Furthermore, even if data from randomized clinical trials do become available, registry data will remain an important resource for monitoring treatment side effects, clinic utilization patterns, characteristics of couples seeking treatment, and changing patterns of service delivery. Therefore, it is essential that the data collected are reliable, valid, and comparable across different registries.

Table 4.5.
OUTCOME DATA REQUIRED FOR REGISTRIES

AREA OF DATA	TOPIC	DATA
Pregnancies	Spontaneous abortion	Weeks of gestation, karyotype anomalies
	Termination of pregnancy	Weeks of gestation
	Ectopic pregnancy	Weeks of gestation
	Birth weight	Grams
	Gestational age	Weeks
	Multiple births	Separate sheet for each baby
	Stillbirth, neonatal death	Weeks of gestation, birth weight, cause of death
	Delivery	Type
	Special care and intensive care	Number of days
	Maternal hospital admission	Antenatal and postnatal length of stay
Women	Death	Cause
	Morbidity (short term)	Postprocedure, puerperium (e.g., hyperstimulation syndrome I, II, III), infection
	Psychological effects	Age
	Cancer incidence	Site, type, age
	Subsequent pregnancy	Reproductive outcomes
	Other disease (e.g., endocrine)	Type, age
Infants and children	Death	Age, cause
	Congenital malformation	Details
	Morbidity	Age, cause
	Cancer	Site, type, age
	Neurodevelopment	Type, age

The choice of data and how it is collected is dictated by the reason for its collection. For the purposes proposed, it is necessary for registries to collect data from individual clinics on the characteristics of women seeking IVF services, the characteristics of women who begin treatment, the treatment employed, and the outcome of treatment including any untoward effects (Table 4.5).

National and regional registries need to include data on every treatment cycle, denoting whether it is the first or subsequent cycle for that particular woman, and the interval since the last cycle. This requires ascertaining whether the couple has been treated previously at other clinics. There should be complete follow-up data recorded on the outcome of pregnancy. The number of new couples beginning treatment each year is an important indicator of the demand for treatment, and national registries also must attempt to obtain data on the long-term outcomes for women and children.

The quality of data collected by registries depends on the quality of record keeping at the clinic level, which varies highly. Record quality is associated with whether the clinic is freestanding or associated with a hospital and whether the couple is referred on after the diagnosis of a clinical pregnancy.

Registry data suffers from a lack of standardization in reporting the outcomes of infertility treatment, including deficiencies in the classification of infertility problems as well as inconsistent methodology. Standard formats for data collection and computerized entry help to assure completeness and accuracy, but even so, certain items may be subject to interpretation. Unambiguous definitions are useful, but a need also exists for educating clinicians regarding form completion and compliance, which in some jurisdictions may now be required by legislation.

RECORD LINKAGE FOR EPIDEMIOLOGICAL INVESTIGATIONS

Many countries have routine birth and death registration. The data collected vary but often include social, demographic, obstetric, and infant outcome data on all pregnancies from 20 weeks of gestation onward. Similarly, many countries also have death, birth defect, and cancer registration. Some collect hospital morbidity discharge data as well as drug prescription data. Linking records of IVF conceptions to existing perinatal databases would be an efficient and inexpensive way of obtaining long-term follow-up health information on women receiving IVF and their children conceived by this procedure.

CONCLUSIONS

From an epidemiological perspective, the quality of nearly all data presently available on the effectiveness of IVF is lacking in several respects. Different definitions are used. Methodologies are weak. Monitoring of data collection is absent, and little or no follow-up data exist on what happens after the pregnancy is established. To correct this situation, both national and regional registries are needed, and these registries must collaborate to standardize data collection and to encourage record linkage with other registries of relevant outcome data.

Proper quality assurance cannot be secured unless such registries include all IVF centers in a given population. In countries where voluntary registration of treatment results in less than 100% participation, governments need to make participation mandatory if the quality of care provided to infertile people is to be assured and meaningful data available for evaluating the new reproductive technologies.

REFERENCES

1. Chillik CF, Acosta AA, Garcia JF, et al. The role of IVF in infertile patients with endometriosis. Fertil Steril 1985;44:56–61.
2. Yovich JL, Yovich JM, Tuvich AL, et al. In vitro fertilization for endometriosis. Lancet 1985;ii:552.
3. Haan G. Health services for infertility: a cost effectiveness analysis from the Netherlands. Paper presented at the WHO-EURO Confer-

ence on the Place of In Vitro Fertilization in Infertility Care. Copenhagen, June 1990.

4. National Perinatal Statistics Unit and the Fertility Society of Australia. IVF and GIFT pregnancies in Australia and New Zealand, 1988. National Perinatal Statistics Unit, Sydney, 1990.

5. The Medical Research Council and the Royal College of Obstetricians and Gynecologists. The Fourth Report of the Voluntary Licensing Authority for Human In Vitro Fertilisation and Embryology. London, 1989.

6. Medical Research International and the Society of Assisted Reproductive Technology of the American Fertility Society. In vitro fertilization/embryo transfer in the United States: 1987 results from the National IVF-ET Registry. Fertil Steril 1989;51:14–19.

7. Wagner MG, St. Clair PA. Are in vitro fertilisation and embryo transfer of benefit to all? Lancet 1989;ii:1027–1030.

8. Tulandi T, Cherry N. Clinical trials in reproductive surgery: randomization and life-table analysis. Fertil Steril 1989;52:12–14.

9. Leridon H, Spira A. Problems in measuring the effectiveness of infertility therapy. Fertil Steril 1984;41:580–586.

10. Cramer DW, Walker AM, Schiff I. Statistical methods in evaluating the outcome of infertility therapy. Fertil Steril 1979;32:80–86.

11. Olive DL. Analysis of fertility trials: a methodologic review. Fertil Steril 1986;45:157–171.

12. Jansen R. The clinical impact of IVF: part 1. Results and limitations of conventional reproductive medicine. Med J Aust 1987;146:342–353.

5

The Financial Costs of
In Vitro Fertilization:
An Example from Australia
■

DITTA BARTELS

In Australia, 7.5% of the gross national product is spent on medical care.[1] Over the last 10 years, this expenditure has remained relatively stable, even though a variety of high-cost medical technologies and procedures have been introduced. The resulting competition for available resources between high-technology medicine on the one hand and routine primary health services on the other has created severe shortages and stresses within the health care system, particularly in services to disabled and elderly people.[1] In this situation, which is by no means unique to Australia, there is an obvious need to assess the public sector costs of the new high-technology medical procedures, including IVF and related technologies.

The debate in Australia as to how it will fund IVF has been ongoing. The public has expressed considerable concern over the costs of IVF technology in light of its rapid expansion and limited benefit to infertile couples. Governments base their funding decisions (at least in part) on estimates of the actual cost of a health service, but in the case of IVF, such estimates are lacking. This point was made explicitly by the Committee of Inquiry into IVF created by the Australian Family Law Council:

Both reproductive technology and technological conceptions are only made possible through the allocation of substantial resources by the community. . . . Despite extensive enquiries, this Committee has been unable to elicit any accurate figures as to the cost to the public purse of reproductive technology research and programmes.[2]

This chapter calculates the cost of a typical IVF treatment cycle and the proportion of this cost borne directly by the Australian government. Furthermore, it estimates the number of IVF treatment cycles performed in Australia during a 5-year period (1980 to 1984) as well as the total direct government expenditure for these services.

DIRECT GOVERNMENT EXPENDITURE IN AUSTRALIA, 1980–1984

A study was conducted in 1987 to estimate the costs of IVF treatment to the government of Australia,[1] where patients pay for a particular item of medical treatment and the government reimburses a proportion of that amount. Private insurance schemes exist that bridge the gap, but because they receive no government support, they do not concern this discussion.

The amounts of reimbursement for various items are set out in the Medicare Benefits Schedule.[3] (The amounts used here are for 1987 and are in Australian dollars.) For example, a clinic visit to a gynecologist is listed as Schedule item #94, with a scheduled fee of A$23.50 and a rebate of A$20. An IVF treatment cycle has no specific item number, but many of the separate steps do as they also are used during other types of gynecological or obstetric care.

The IVF treatment cycle was divided in the 1987 study into four stages: prelaparoscopy, laparoscopy, fertilization in vitro, and the embryo transfer and assessment of pregnancy. For each stage, the various separate items of expenditure together with their Schedule item number, scheduled fee, and government rebate were listed. Table 5.1 shows a detailed breakdown for the prelaparoscopy stage.

It should be noted that the treatment steps presented in Table 5.1 refer to a much earlier stage in the development of IVF technology than we deal with today. Hospitalization, for example, is no longer common, and this can reduce the cost of treatment substantially. Monitoring of ovulation by hormonal means also has been replaced to a large extent by ultrasound evaluation. Still, while the details of Table 5.1 are no longer up-to-date, the methodology continues to be useful for countries with a system of reimbursement similar to that in Australia.

Table 5.2 details the later treatment stages, from the recovery of ripe eggs to the assessment of pregnancy. The main difference between the early 1980s and today is that laparoscopy has given way to egg retrieval by ultrasound-guided techniques.

Table 5.1.
COSTS ASSOCIATED WITH IVF PRELAPAROSCOPY STAGE

TREATMENT	No.	COST, A$ Unit	COST, A$ Total	GOVERNMENTAL CONTRIBUTION, A$ Unit	GOVERNMENTAL CONTRIBUTION, A$ Total
Superovulation					
Pergonal	20	14.00	280.00	14.00	280.00
Clomid	2	26.00	52.00	1.00	2.00
Consultations	6	23.50	141.00	20.00	120.00
Monitoring					
Estradiol	8	42.75	342.00	36.35	291.00
Luteinizing hormone	11	25.90	285.00	22.05	243.00
Progesterone	7	25.90	181.00	22.05	154.00
Ultrasound	2	102.00	204.00	86.00	172.00
Gonadex	—	—	20.00	—	20.00
Semen analysis	1	25.90	26.00	22.05	22.00
Hospitalization	5	230.00	1,150.00	125.00	625.00
Total			**2,681.00**		**1,929.00**

Sources: Expenditures are calculated in 1987 prices and based on information supplied by the Australian Department of Health.

Table 5.2.
COSTS OF IVF TREATMENTS FROM LAPAROSCOPY
STAGE TO ASSESSMENT OF PREGNANCY

TREATMENT	COST, A$	GOVERNMENTAL CONTRIBUTION, A$
Laparoscopy		
Surgeon	225.00	205.00
Anesthetist	65.00	55.00
Fertilization	500.00	250.00
Embryo transfer	47.00	40.00
Assessment of pregnancy		
Luteinizing hormone	26.00	22.00
Progesterone	26.00	22.00
Estradiol	43.00	36.00
Consultation	23.00	20.00
Ultrasound	102.00	86.00
Total	**1,057.00**	**736.00**

Sources: See Table 5.1.

The actual step of fertilization in vitro does not have a Schedule item number. To have brought this particular item into the Australian Medicare system would have required a political decision by the government signaling all-out acceptance of IVF, and as late as the end of 1988, the Australian Federal Government was not prepared to take that step. Actually, IVF providers exerted little pressure on the government to do so, because all of the treatment stages other than fertilization in vitro were covered by Medicare anyway. Also, an effective way was found to receive payment for the fertilization procedure without imposing a great burden on individual patients: patients simply were requested to make a tax-deductible donation to the IVF research unit affiliated with the IVF clinic. Donations generally were set between A$500 and A$800, so considering the Australian marginal tax rate was

50% during the early 1980s, the indirect government contribution to the fertilization procedure by this method was approximately A$250.

In total, the costs for a single IVF treatment were A$3,738, with a direct contribution by the government of A$2,665. Therefore, the Australian Federal Government pays for some 70% of the direct cost of an IVF treatment.

NUMBER OF TREATMENTS PERFORMED IN AUSTRALIA, 1980–1984

In 1986, an Australian IVF team at Monash University published its cumulative data on the pregnancy rates achieved during the 5-year period of 1980 to 1984.[4] In their series, 1,775 treatments were performed during this time, resulting in 229 clinical pregnancies (i.e., pregnancies diagnosed by a rise in blood hormone levels following IVF treatment). Therefore, the ratio of treatment cycles to pregnancies was 7.75 to 1. The Monash team did not report how many of these early pregnancies actually led to live births, but information of this kind has become available in aggregated form for all Australia through the National Perinatal Statistics Unit.[5,6]

The report published by this Unit in 1985[5] covered the period of 1980 to 1984, and it included cumulative data on 11 IVF centers. At that time, the Perinatal Statistics Unit did not supply data on the number of treatment cycles performed in the various centers. Rather, data were given only in terms of clinical pregnancies and their outcomes. Altogether, 909 clinical pregnancies had been achieved in Australia during the period considered, but all of these by no means resulted in the birth of live babies, as shown in Table 5.3.

By relating the data in Table 5.3 to that provided in the Monash IVF Center study, cost calculations could be undertaken. At the Monash University IVF Center, 1,775 treatment cycles produced 229 hormonally defined pregnancies, yielding a ratio of

Table 5.3.
OUTCOMES FOLLOWING IVF TREATMENTS,
1979–1984

Hormonally defined pregnancies	909
Pregnancies resulting in live births	496
Unsuccessful outcomes	413
Preclinical abortions	174
Ectopic pregnancies	45
Abortions before 20 weeks	172
Stillbirths	22

Source: National Perinatal Statistics Unit of Australia.

7.75 IVF treatment cycles to 1 hormonally defined pregnancy. During the period of 1980 to 1984, a total of 909 hormonally defined pregnancies were recorded in all of Australia; with the ratio achieved by the Monash Center of 7.75 to 1, this would mean that 7,045 treatment cycles would have been required to yield the 909 hormonally defined pregnancies recorded for that period. Monash University, however, was by far the most successful IVF center in Australia in hormonal superovulation and monitoring, egg collection, fertilization in vitro, and embryo culture. It stands to reason that the other, less successful IVF centers had ratios of treatment cycles to hormonally defined pregnancies that were greater than 7.75 to 1. In turn, this would mean that considerably more than 7,045 IVF treatment cycles would have been needed in the 5-year period to yield the 909 hormonally defined pregnancies recorded. Unfortunately, no IVF center in Australia other than Monash had reported its success rates by 1987, so cost estimates were based on the assumption that, on average, approximately twice as many treatment cycles per hormonally defined pregnancy were required in the other IVF programs as at the Monash Center. This would lead to approximately 12,000 treatment cycles performed in Australia during that 5-year period. Given that the direct contribution of the government for one IVF treatment cycle is A$2,665, approximately A$32 million in total were spent by the Australian government for IVF treatments from 1980 to 1984.

COSTS OF HIGH-RISK PREGNANCIES AND NEONATES

Approximately 25% of all IVF pregnancies are multiple pregnancies.[7] Among these, 15% are triplets or quadruplets.[7] The management of multiple pregnancies and births, especially triplets and quadruplets, is quite expensive, because they often are born either too soon or too small. Table 5.4 shows the numbers of very-low-birth-weight babies born in Australia as a result of IVF and GIFT treatments performed in 1986.

In Australia, all babies born weighing 1,500 g or less are placed in neonatal intensive care units. The average costs incurred for the care of babies less than 1,000 g is A$72,000 per baby; the average cost for the care of babies between 1,000 and 1,500 g is A$25,000 per baby.[8] These estimates also can be applied to the IVF and GIFT birth cohort of 1986 (Table 5.5).

The intensive care of IVF and GIFT babies, therefore, costs

Table 5.4.
VERY-LOW-BIRTH-WEIGHT ASSISTED-CONCEPTION
BABIES CONCEIVED IN 1986

BIRTH WEIGHT, g	BABIES, n		
	IVF	GIFT	Total
< 1,000	24	16	40
1,000–1,500	34	14	48
Total	**58**	**30**	**88**

Source: National Perinatat Statistics Unit of Australia.

Table 5.5.
NEONATAL INTENSIVE CARE COSTS FOR IVF AND GIFT BABIES
CONCEIVED IN 1986

BIRTH WEIGHT, g	COST PER BABY, A$	BABIES, n	TOTAL COST, A$
< 1,000	72,000	40	2.9 million
1,000–1,500	25,000	48	1.2 million
Total		88	4.1 million

Source: Henderson-Smart 1988.[9]

the Australian government approximately A$4 million per year. This figure is in addition to the A$32 million in direct costs for IVF treatment spent by the government during the period of 1980 to 1984. By 1987, the direct annual cost to the government was A$17 million.[10]

Very-low-birth-weight babies also are born in normal pregnancies, but the rate in both IVF and GIFT pregnancies is a great deal higher. In 1986, 11.6% of all Australian IVF babies were very low birth weight (< 1,500 g), whereas in 1985, only 1% of all babies born in the State of Victoria were of very low birth weight.[8] The availability of cots in neonatal intensive care units is based on the occurrence of low-birth-weight babies in the general population; with a rate 11 times higher than in the general population, low-birth-weight IVF and GIFT babies are straining neonatal intensive care facilities. It is not only a question of A$4.1 million having to be spent on this care, but also that the required facilities are then not available to cope with the extra influx of very-low-birth-weight IVF and GIFT babies.

CONCLUSIONS

Clearly, the financial contribution of the Australian government to IVF programs is considerable, and it is not limited to the direct costs of IVF treatment. These estimates do not include the cost of long-term care for babies born under 1,000 g, who have a 20% to 30% chance of permanent sensory, cognitive, or motor impairment.[9] Similarly, no attempt is made to estimate the costs to the community of high-risk pregnancy care for the mothers of IVF babies.

The proliferation of IVF services in Australia since the early 1980s has important implications both for health and for health care cost containment. Between 1980 and 1984, an estimated 12,000 treatment cycles were performed (an average of 2,400 treatment cycles per year), but over 8,300 treatment cycles were performed during 1987 alone. Therefore, as a component of overall health care expenditures, the burgeoning IVF enterprise is no longer an insignificant part.

The extent to which the Australian system of health care financing itself has encouraged the proliferation of IVF services is unclear. In Australia, where the government pays 70% of the treatment cost, 519 treatments per million inhabitants occurred during 1987. In Britain, where the National Health Service pays for only a fraction of IVF treatments and the rest are paid for by the clients themselves, only 117 treatments per million inhabitants occurred the year before.[11] This may mean that IVF consumption is highly sensitive to price, which strongly suggests that IVF is a discretionary—rather than an essential—health service.

It is important to consider this when planning for the health service needs of a nation. Essential health services that benefit many people, such as primary care for pregnant women, children, and the elderly, should not be forced to make due with shrinking resources in favor of expensive, high-technology treatments such as IVF that benefit only a few. Furthermore, the costs must be calculated to include both the direct and the indirect costs, and these true costs must not be hidden from the government and the public. These true costs must be available for the purposes of priority setting and policy decisions.

REFERENCES

1. Bartels D. Government expenditure on IVF programs: an exploratory study. Prometheus 1987;5:304–324.

2. Family Law Council. Creating Children. Canberra: Australian Government Printing Services, 1985:4, 19.
3. Department of Health. Medicare Benefits Schedule Book. Canberra: Australian Government Printing Services, 1986.
4. Kovacs GT, Rogers P, Leeton JF, et al. In vitro fertilisation and embryo transfer: prospects of pregnancy by life-table analysis. Med J Aust 1986;144:682–683.
5. National Perinatal Statistics Unit and Fertility Society of Australia. In Vitro Fertilization Pregnancies Australia and New Zealand, 1979–1984. Sydney: National Perinatal Statistics Unit, 1985.
6. National Perinatal Statistics Unit and Fertility Society of Australia. In Vitro Fertilization Pregnancies Australia and New Zealand, 1979–1985. Sydney: National Perinatal Statistics Unit, 1987.
7. National Perinatal Statistics Unit and Fertility Society of Australia. IVF and GIFT Pregnancies Australia and New Zealand, 1986. Sydney: National Perinatal Statistics Unit, 1987.
8. Consultative Council on Obstetric and Paediatric Mortality and Morbidity. Annual Report for the Year 1985. Melbourne: Consultative Council, 1986.
9. Henderson-Smart DJ. Neonatal intensive-care—where to draw the line? Presented at the ANZAAS Centenary Congress, University of Sydney, May 1988.
10. Department of Community Services and Health. In Vitro Fertilisation in Australia. Canberra: Department of Community Services and Health, 1988.
11. Voluntary Licensing Authority for Human In Vitro Fertilisation and Embryology. The Third Report. London: Voluntary Licensing Authority, 1988.

6

Health Services for Infertility: A Cost-Effectiveness Analysis from the Netherlands

■

GER HAAN

For several years, Dutch health authorities have had a policy of deferred adoption of new medical technologies in the social health insurance package. During a trial period, the new technology is provided on a limited basis, under defined conditions, and data collected for a cost-effectiveness analysis. One of the first technologies to be evaluated under this system was IVF; the decision on its inclusion in the social package was to be postponed until the results of the evaluation were available.

The evaluation was conducted by researchers at the University of Limburg, and it was financed by the Health Insurance Executive Board (Ziekenfondsraad), which is the advisory board to the Dutch government on behalf of the social insurers. The Health Insurance Executive Board raised several questions, including whether IVF should be included in the social insurance package given the costs and effects of treatment, and how IVF compared with alternative medical treatments for infertility.

Data from five Dutch IVF centers (Dijkzigt Hospital, Rotterdam; Free University Hospital, Amsterdam; Academic Hospital, Leiden; St. Radboud Hospital, Nijmegen; and St. Elisabeth Hospital, Tilburg) were collected between August 1986 and June 1988.

All women beginning treatment during this period ($n = 1,462$) were included in the study. Many received more than one treatment, so data arc available from 3,092 IVF treatment cycles. Comparison with other infertility treatments was based on a review of the literature.

SUCCESS RATES

Because IVF treatment is a chain of several individual phases, success rates can be presented in several ways. Figure 6.1 illustrates the drop-out rate per treatment phase. Approximately 20% of stimulation cycles fail to reach the follicle aspiration stage, and another 10% fail to reach the embryo-transfer stage. Of treatment cycles reaching the embryo-transfer stage, 20% result in a clinical pregnancy. The take-at-least-one-baby-home rate per started IVF treatment cycle is only 10%, which agrees with population-based registry data from Australia, New Zealand,[1] the United Kingdom,[2] and the United States.[3]

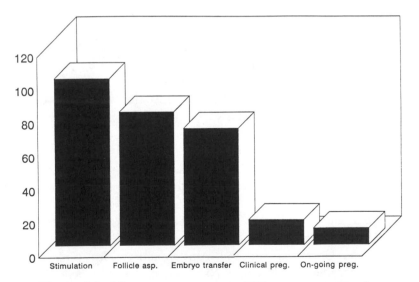

Figure 6.1. Mean success rate per IVF treatment episode.

Clinical pregnancy losses were mainly accounted for by spontaneous abortion (17%) or extrauterine pregnancy (6%). Thirty percent of ongoing pregnancies were multiple, which was one reason for the higher than expected number of pregnancy and perinatal complications in this evaluation. The complication rate, however, also was elevated for single pregnancies; whether characteristics of the IVF population or aspects of the treatment itself caused this could not be determined. Six of 393 children (1.5%) had congenital malformations, of which two cases (0.5%) were anencephaly.

Of course, a 10% success rate is not very high, but 10% is the success rate per IVF treatment cycle. A failed treatment cycle can be followed by another attempt; therefore, cumulative pregnancy rates also were calculated using two methods.

First, a cumulative, ongoing pregnancy rate was calculated for a specified number of treatment cycles, using women rather than treatment cycles as the unit of analysis. Projected (estimated) success rates were based on actual success rates per treatment cycle. After the first IVF treatment, 12% of the women achieved an ongoing pregnancy. With continuation to three treatments after earlier failures, this estimate increased to almost 30%. With continuation to six treatments, the cumulative, ongoing pregnancy rate increased to 42%. Most couples, however, are not prepared to continue for so many cycles.

Second, cumulative pregnancy rates also were derived using a cohort approach. A total of 852 couples were followed for at least 1 year after their first IVF treatment, and almost 25% of the women achieved an ongoing pregnancy, with an average of 2.5 started treatments and two follicle aspirations.

TREATMENT RESULTS

As expected, IVF was most successful in those instances when a good follicular growth phase was established, resulting in mature oocytes. If these oocytes were fertilized in vitro with good-quality sperm, then a reasonable chance for fertilization and embryo development existed. Pregnancy rates strongly depended on both the number and quality of the embryos transferred.

Beyond this simple clinical analysis, success rates differed markedly among both patient groups and hospitals. The differences found in univariate analyses were confirmed by a multivariate, logistic regression model in which both patient and hospital variables were included as independent variables.

Success rates were reduced when a male factor was involved or when the woman had only one ovary. Couples with a long history of infertility (6 years or more) were less likely to succeed with IVF, as were women over 40 years of age.

Success rates among hospitals differed by a factor of 2.5, even after correction for differences in the patient case-mix. The influence of several treatment factors (stimulation regimen, time between treatments, and type of follicle aspiration) was minimal.

COSTS

Calculations of the real costs of IVF treatment were based on assessments of the personnel, equipment, and materials needed to run an IVF program of a specific size. Most of the cost items (apart from materials and drugs) were fixed, and they related only to the size of the program. This is the consequence of an important characteristic of IVF programs: the so-called "availability utility." This means that personnel, equipment, and locations must be available even though they might not be performing IVF activities at all times. Therefore, cost calculations are based mainly on capacity assumptions for personnel, equipment, and locations.

Total treatment costs for an IVF program were expressed as the average cost per started treatment. The average cost per started treatment was lower than the cost of a completed treatment (including embryo transfer and luteal phase support), and the cost of the IVF treatment depended highly on:

1. The treatment protocol (medication and frequency of both hormonal and ultrasound monitoring)

2. The task division between academic and other personnel. The ultimate responsibility for IVF activities rests with a gynecologist or biologist; however, the execution of procedures may be delegated to other qualified personnel—medical doctors and nurses
3. The organization's planning and structuring of activities
4. The size of the IVF program
5. Physician's fees

For an IVF program of 375 started treatments annually, the average cost per started treatment was between NLG (Dutch guilders) 2,600 and 3,300 (NLG 1 = US $0.50) (Figure 6.2). The average cost per started treatment was NLG 2,100 to 2,700 for a program of 750 treatments and NLG 2,000 to 2,400 for a program of 1,250 treatments.

These data imply that programs of approximately 750 started treatments per year are more efficient than smaller programs. Up to a certain break point, larger IVF programs can be managed by

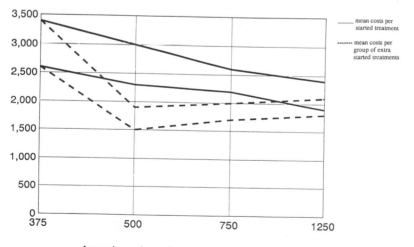

Figure 6.2. Mean versus differential costs (in Dutch guilders) in relation to the annual number of IVF treatments per center.

more or less the same group of professionals and the same equipment as needed for a smaller program. In other words, the costs for both personnel and equipment are semifixed in relation to the size of the program; they grow stepwise with extension of the program.

Hospital-scale efficiency cannot be improved further by expanding the program beyond an annual 750 treatments, but on a national scale, it is much more efficient to have only a few hospitals with very large programs than a large number of hospitals with smaller programs, as Table 6.1 illustrates. A national IVF program with an annual number of 3,000 started treatments would be 20% less expensive if carried out in four instead of eight centers.

COST-EFFECTIVENESS

The ultimate goal of IVF treatment is the birth of a baby. If the average cost per started treatment is set at NLG 2,500, then the average treatment cost per achieved full-term pregnancy is NLG 25,000, based on a 10% success rate per started treatment. Including the additional health care costs of the pregnancy and prenatal care, the average costs increase to approximately NLG 30,000.

Table 6.1.
TOTAL COSTS FOR A NATIONAL IVF PROGRAM
OF 3,000 STARTED TREATMENTS

OPTION	TOTAL COSTS*
8 centers with 375 treatments each	7.74–10.02
6 centers with 500 treatments each	6.95–8.98
1 center with 1,250, 1 center with 750, 2 centers with 500 treatments each	6.41–8.05

*Costs are in million Dutch guilders.

Table 6.2.
DIFFERENTIATED TREATMENT COSTS
PER ONGOING PREGNANCY*

Patient groups	
Only tubal pathology	22,000
Male factor	43,000
One ovary (two ovaries)	33,000 (22,000)
Woman > 35 years (≤ 35)	36,000 (21,000)
Infertility period > 5 years	30,000
Primary infertility (secondary)	27,000 (20,000)
Maximum number of treatments	
1	20,000
3	23,000 (24,000 for treatment episodes 2 and 3)
6	27,000 (38,000 for treatment episodes 4 to 6)
IVF center	
Best	17,000
Worst	48,000
Annual number of IVF treatments per center	
375	26,000 to 33,000
500	23,000 to 30,000 (15,000 to 20,000 for the additional 125)
750	21,000 to 27,000 (17,000 to 20,000 for the additional 250)
1250	20,000 to 24,000 (17,000 to 20,000 for the additional 500)

*The average costs (in Dutch guilders) per reached ongoing pregnancy were 25,000.

Averages, however, mask the differences in costs involved in achieving the same outcome between patient groups, hospitals, number of treatments per couple, and the size of IVF programs, as Table 6.2 illustrates. Average treatment costs per started treatment differ little among patient groups, but the average treatment costs per achieved full-term pregnancy do. For example, the treatment costs per ongoing pregnancy where the indication for IVF is a male factor amount to almost NLG 43,000; for other patient groups with relatively low success rates (women with one ovary, older women), this figure is between NLG 30,000 and 35,000.

The average IVF treatment costs per achieved full-term pregnancy are NLG 20,000 for only one treatment. If couples undergo a second or third treatment after earlier failures, then the average costs per achieved full-term pregancy grow to NLG 24,000 for the second and third treatment cycles. This means that the average costs per achieved full-term pregnancy for the first three treatments together are NLG 22,500; the average costs per achieved full-term pregnancy when four to six cycles are required is almost NLG 38,000. For reasons of both efficiency and equity, limiting the number of treatment cycles per couple should be considered.

Regarding treatment costs per achieved full-term pregnancy in relation to the size of the IVF program, the costs per achieved pregnancy in a program of 375 treatments per year are approximately one-third higher than in a program of 1,250 treatments per year (NLG 26,000 to 33,000 v. NLG 20,000 to 24,000).

OTHER INFERTILITY TREATMENTS

The cost-effectiveness of IVF also was compared with tubal surgery in this evaluation, because tubal surgery always has been paid for by the government in the Netherlands. Tubal pathology was commonplace among the study population as well. The average success rate (expressed as the percentage achieving an ongoing pregnancy) after tubal surgery is approximately 30%,[4] with a range of 0% to 75% depending on the type and extent of tubal damage. Tubal surgery has decided advantages over IVF in that it might restore fertility.

The treatment cost per tubal surgery is between NLG 5,000 and 7,000. If additional health care costs related to tubal surgery (especially for treatment of extrauterine pregnancy) are included, then these figures increase by approximately 10%, to NLG 5,500 and 7,700. Based on an average ongoing pregnancy rate of 30%, the average treatment costs per achieved ongoing pregnancy by tubal surgery are approximately NLG 17,000 to 23,000.

On average, three IVF treatments are needed to reach an ongoing pregnancy rate of 30%. The average costs per ongoing pregnancy when three IVF treatments are required is approximately NLG 22,500, approximately equivalent to the cost of one reconstructive operation. Results differ greatly among patient groups, however, both for IVF and tubal surgery. In terms of efficiency, some patient groups are better off with IVF; others are better off with tubal surgery. Clearly, both options should be available, and the choice of treatment should be made on the basis of the prognosis for a given patient seeking treatment rather than on the conditions of physical or financial accessibility.

CONCLUSIONS

Several results of this study have important health policy implications, both for the Netherlands and elsewhere. Most population-based data currently available from IVF registries count events per started treatment, per embryo-transfer cycle, or per oocyte-retrieval cycle. To date, no information has been available on the series of events for a cohort of women entering treatment. By using this cohort approach, one can obtain accurate cumulative effectiveness rates, estimates of the percentages of women dropping out of treatment after each phase, and information on the variations in effectiveness rates according to the size of an IVF program and the cause of infertility. These data make clear that some IVF centers are better than others, even after adjusting for case-mix. Furthermore, larger IVF centers are more efficient (up to a point) than smaller centers, but most importantly, these data demonstrate the fallacy of the popular notion that cumulative "success" rates are additive, that is, that the probability of success with one IVF attempt is 10% and with six attempts is 60%. Cumulative success rates are not linear; after three cycles of treatment, the likelihood of success falls as the cost to achieve a pregnancy rises. There is good scientific justification, therefore, to limit the number of treatment cycles to no more than three.

Regarding the policy decision taken in the Netherlands, the Health Insurance Executive Board finally decided after lengthy debate to advise the Dutch Ministry of Health to create a reimbursement situation that provided equal geographical and financial accessibility for IVF in comparison with other infertility treatments. Information about the cost-effectiveness of IVF in relation to other infertility treatments, however, hardly had any influence on the final decision about public financing for IVF. In part, this was because the entire structure of health care insurance had come into discussion in the Netherlands during the time of the study, and the discussion of IVF financing was overshadowed by that of if and how to finance all health care services. The "IVF question" that initially was a comparison between IVF and other infertility treatments evolved into a discussion of the merits of infertility treatment versus other health care services. The central question was whether to include IVF and other infertity services within the base insurance or an optional benefits package.

In 1985, the Dutch Ministry of Health announced that IVF programs would be licensed by the government pending the results of the cost-effectiveness study. At the study's completion, reliable and detailed data were available on which to base a decision concerning licensing, but no such decision was forthcoming. In 1989, a new regulatory announcement was made: the number of IVF laboratories would be limited to 10. At that moment, however, 14 laboratories were involved in IVF. The initial limit was raised to 11, and then finally 12 laboratories were given permission to continue their activities. They also were free to choose the number of transport IVF centers with which to collaborate. (The number of transport IVF centers is approximately 30.) The decision was one of political convenience in that following the recommendation of the study would require six IVF laboratories to close.

In the Dutch evaluation, no account is made for untoward risks or ethical and legal considerations posed by one treatment versus another. It must be remembered that most medical treatments involve some risks, and unequal availablity and reimbursement for various infertility treatments also pose ethical dilemmas for policy makers. The cost-effectiveness study of IVF in the Netherlands was notable in that it was explicitly linked to policy decisions regarding reimbursement and clinic licensure; nevertheless, the original intent of the government both to regulate and contain service provision was abandoned. This should not imply that technology assessment has no role in rational policy-making. Rather, the links between research and policy-making still are quite weak.

ACKNOWLEDGMENT

I am indebted to all participants of this study for their collaboration, especially Bob Leerentveld, Rob Bernardus, Cees Waegemaekers, Hans Hollanders, and Frederika Prak as representatives of the IVF teams, and Reg van Steen and Frans Rutten as representatives of the Maastricht research group. The study described in this chapter was supported by a grant from the Dutch Health Insurance Executive Board.

REFERENCES

1. National Perinatal Statistic Unit and the Fertility Society of Australia. IVF and GIFT Pregnancies in Australia and New Zealand. Sydney: National Perinatal Statistics Unit, 1990.
2. Medical Research Council and the Royal College of Obstetricians and Gynecologists. The Fourth Report of the Voluntary Licensing Authority for Human In Vitro Fertilisation and Embryology. London: Medical Research Council and Royal College of Obstetricians and Gynecologists, 1989.
3. Medical Research Institute and the Society of Assisted Reproductive Technology of the American Fertility Society. In Vitro Fertilization/Embryo Transfer in the United States: 1987 Results from the National IVF/ET Registry. Fertil Steril 1987;51:14–19.
4. Soules MR. Infertility surgery. In: DeCherney AH, ed. Reproductive Failure. New York: Churchill Livingstone, 1986.

PART III

RISK ASSESSMENT

7

Ovulation Induction During Treatment of Infertility: An Assessment of the Risks

■

PATRICIA STEPHENSON

Inducing ovulation involves stimulating the ovaries with chemical preparations (so-called "fertility drugs") to encourage the maturation of multiple ovarian follicles. Ovulation induction may be used as a medical treatment of infertility or as a preparatory step for artificial insemination or IVF. This chapter discusses the safety of two drugs commonly used to induce ovulation: clomiphene citrate and human menopausal gonadotropin (hMG).

Clomiphene citrate is a synthetic, nonsteroidal, triphenylethylene compound;[1,2] hMG is a purified extract of human female urine containing both follicle-stimulating and luteinizing hormone.[1,2]

The predominant medical opinion holds that clomiphene citrate and hMG are safe and effective but that serious side effects sometimes do occur. This presumption of safety must be regarded with measured skepticism. By current standards, both clomiphene citrate and hMG were never evaluated properly before their introduction into clinical practice; even today, nearly 30 years later, methodologically sound research is still lacking. Widespread use of these drugs has led health policy makers, researchers, and the public to voice concerns about the risks of ovulation induction.

METHODS AND MATERIALS

A literature search of the Medline bibliographic database and Shepard's Catalog of Teratogenic Agents was conducted.[3] This was followed by a manual search. Book chapters, abstracts, and other non—peer-reviewed publications were excluded from this review, and a special effort was made to locate studies that reported negative findings.

A distinction is made between "known" and "suspected" adverse effects. Known adverse effects are those for which evidence exists of a direct association between ovulation induction and the adverse effect in question. Suspected adverse effects are those for which the evidence leaves room for doubt.

Different types of evidence are presented, including experimental studies, case reports, clinical case series, population-based series, and case-control studies. Each type of evidence has both strengths and weaknesses to consider when evaluating the likelihood that a reported association is real.

Experimental studies using animal models or genetic materials test hypotheses regarding the biological effects of ovulation induction. Evidence from such studies is inconclusive, however, because interspecies biological variability cannot be ruled out.

Case reports of adverse effects occurring in one or more women undergoing treatment are useful in generating hypotheses. Still, these merely suggest the possibility that an association exists; they do not offer proof.

Clinical case series provide information on the incidence of adverse effects in clinical populations undergoing treatment. In large series, these data may be compared with the expected incidence in the general population. Such studies do not provide evidence for a direct association, because no attempt is made to control for the confounding effects of maternal characteristics or preexisting health conditions.

Population-based series combine data from several clinics that serve a particular geographical area (usually a country). These studies are better sources of information from which to compare the incidence of adverse effects among women receiving treatment with the expected incidence in the general population. The bias resulting from referral patterns and self-selection into particular clinic populations is eliminated, but even so, adequate control for confounding factors is not achieved.

Case-control studies compare women diagnosed as having a condition (thought to be an adverse effect of treatment) with women who do not have that condition. The purpose here is to determine if the two groups differ in the proportion of women exposed to ovulation induction drugs either before or during pregnancy. Again, available studies do not adequately control for factors that could increase a woman's probability both of exposure to ovulation induction and of having the condition in question.

Case reports, clinical case series, and population-based series can provide conclusive evidence for a direct association between ovulation induction and adverse pregnancy outcome when certain conditions are met. There must be a known biological mechanism to explain the association. Also, the adverse effect must not (or only rarely) occur in the absence of drug exposure, and cases of the adverse effect following drug exposure must be reported in several different clinical populations.

KNOWN ADVERSE EFFECTS

Multiple pregnancy

Ovulation induction greatly increases the risk of multiple gestation. Even with improved ovulation induction protocols and intensive monitoring, it is not possible to control precisely the number of ovarian follicles and oocytes that develop.[4] When ovulation induction is used in conjunction with IVF, the likelihood of pregnancy depends on the number of embryos transferred.[5] This has encouraged the practice of transferring three or more embryos per treatment attempt,[5] and the probability of a multiple pregnancy increases with the number of embryos transferred.[5]

Multiple-pregnancy rates after ovulation induction reported in case series range from 8% to 13% when clomiphene citrate is used[6] and from 9% to 42% with hMG.[6,7] Population-based series from Great Britain,[8] the United States,[9] and Australia and New Zealand[10] report multiple-pregnancy rates of approximately 25% for IVF births. The expected incidence of multiple pregnancy in the general population is approximately 1% to 2%.[11,12]

Pregnancy wastage

Perinatal mortality is high among babies born after treatment for infertility. In large part, this is because of the increased frequency of multiple pregnancy. Multiple births tend to be premature, and those premature babies who survive are at increased risk for major neurological handicap, cerebral palsy, mental retardation, and sensory impairments.[13]

Perinatal mortality rates after ovulation induction, calculated from data reported in case series, range from 0.0 to 262.3.[14–33] When the data from the various studies are combined, the perinatal mortality rate is 45.2 per 1,000 live births and fetal deaths. This rate is two to three times higher than the perinatal mortality rates in the general population for the same countries during similar periods.[34]

Perinatal mortality is no less a problem for IVF pregnancies. A recent population-based series of IVF births in Great Britain reported a perinatal mortality rate of 27.2.[8] A similar study from Australia and New Zealand reported a perinatal mortality rate of 44.2.[10] These rates are three and four times higher than the rates for the general population in the respective countries.

Ovarian hyperstimulation

The ovarian hyperstimulation syndrome is another important iatrogenic consequence in treatment of infertility. It is characterized by a marked increase in vascular permeability and the rapid accumulation of fluid in the peritoneal, pleural, and pericardial cavities. This in turn may lead to hypovolemia, hemoconcentration, electrolyte imbalance, ascites, hemoperitoneum, pleural effusion, hydrothorax, acute pulmonary distress, thromboembolism, thrombophlebitis, pulmonary embolism, stroke, arterial occlusion necessitating limb amputation, atelectasis, or death.[17,18,35–59]

While there are several case reports of severe ovarian hyperstimulation syndrome with clomiphene citrate,[50–54] this syndrome is more common, severe, and protracted with hMG or hMG combined with other drugs.[1,2] In case series, the modal incidence of the severe form is approximately 1% to 2%.[7,35] Ovarian hyperstimulation syndrome is extremely rare following natural conception.

SUSPECTED ADVERSE EFFECTS

Extrauterine pregnancy

Extrauterine pregnancy (ectopic or heterotopic pregnancy) may be another serious side effect in treatment of infertility. Several explanations exist for the increased incidence of extrauterine pregnancy in women receiving such treatment. Tubal adhesions, a cause of infertility, increase the risk of ectopic pregnancy,[60] and it also has been suggested that the probability of ectopic pregnancy increases according to the number of ovulations.[60] Additionally, the high estrogen levels resulting from treatment with fertility drugs may cause "tubal locking," wherein the ovum becomes isolated in a particular segment of the fallopian tube as a consequence of dysfunctional tubal contractions.[60] The techniques used during IVF for embryo transfer also may be associated with ectopic pregnancy.[61]

At least 49 cases of heterotopic pregnancy associated with ovulation induction either alone or with IVF have been reported.[61–83] Abdominal, cervical, and bilateral tubal pregnancies have been reported as well.[84–86] The incidence of heterotopic pregnancy in induced pregnancies is estimated at 1 in 100,[70,72] whereas in the general population it is estimated at 1 in 3,000 to 1 in 8,000 pregnancies.[87–89]

Several case series reported the incidence of ectopic pregnancies after ovulation induction to be 0.5% to 4.6%.[15,16,19,20,27,46,60–62,90] Others did not mention ectopic pregnancy as a treatment outcome.[14,17,18,21–26,28–33,91]

The incidence of ectopic pregnancy following IVF is more consistent across population-based series, ranging from 5.2% to 7.0%.[9,10,92] The incidence of ectopic pregnancy in the general population is approximately 1%.[62,93]

One population-based, case-control study found that the risk for ectopic pregnancy was elevated ten-fold (95% CI, 1.8, 56.8) among women who had used clomiphene citrate during the index pregnancy.[94] The majority of exposed women at the time of surgery were found to have pelvic adhesions, so the elevated risk associated with use of clomiphene citrate could be caused by confounding if pelvic adhesions are related to clomiphene citrate therapy.

Congenital anomalies

The hypothesis that ovulation induction may be a risk factor for congenital anomalies is more controversial. Clomiphene citrate has been of particular concern, because it is structurally similar to diethystilbestrol (DES),[1,2] a drug known to cause cancer of the vagina and cervix, infertility, spontaneous abortion, ectopic pregnancy, and premature delivery in some daughters of women who took the drug during pregnancy.[95] Clomiphene citrate is contraindicated during pregnancy, but fetal exposure still can occur. Clomiphene citrate has a long half-life and may be present in the body well into the first trimester.[1,2] It also accumulates at significant levels in women receiving multiple courses of therapy.[1,2] Furthermore, clomiphene citrate sometimes will be given inadvertently to women with established pregnancies.

In rats and rabbits, clomiphene citrate is associated with teratogenic mutations, causing cataracts, hydramnios, gastroschisis, cranioschisis, stunted limbs, cleft palate, and hydrocephalus.[96-98] Limb malformations in mice following exposure to hMG have been reported as well,[99,100] but a replication study using the same species failed to confirm this finding.[101] Several studies demonstrated increased chromosomal aberrations in mouse and rabbit embryos exposed to ovulation-induction agents in utero,[102-107] but negative findings also have been reported.[108,109]

Other studies using animal models support the hypothesis that clomiphene citrate may produce defects similar to those that result from in utero exposure to DES. In rats and mice, clomiphene citrate produces cellular changes in vaginal, uterine, and fallopian tube structures similar to those seen after DES exposure.[110–117] Cunha and coworkers[118] observed the same malformations in human vaginal epithelium grafted to host mice and exposed to low doses of clomiphene citrate.

In humans, clomiphene citrate and hMG significantly increase the incidence of chromosomal abnormalities in the embryo. In a study of 1,500 first-trimester spontaneous abortions, Boué and colleagues[119,120] found that abortuses exposed to ovulation-induction drugs during the cycle in which fertilization occurred or in the cycle before fertilization were similar, with 83% and 86% abnormal karyotypes, repectively. Only 60% of abortuses from women who had not taken drugs and 61% of abortuses from women who had taken drugs two or more cycles before fertilization had abnormal karyotypes. Boué and coworkers concluded that fertility drugs increase the risk of releasing oocytes that carry a chromosomal anomaly.

Clinical evidence is equivocal. Numerous case reports link exposure to clomiphene citrate and hMG with neural tube defects, major cardiac anomalies, congenital absence of kidney, Down syndrome, congenital retinopathy, fetal ovarian cysts and dysplasia, hepatoblastoma, club foot, extropia, blocked tear duct, tibial torsion, hemangioma, syndactyly, hypospadias, microcephaly, cleft lip and palate, and polydactyly.[121–135] In case series, the overall incidence of congenital anomalies in infants exposed either to clomiphene citrate or hMG is no higher than the incidence in the general population.[19–33,136,137]

In the population-based series of IVF births in Great Britain[8] and Australia and New Zealand,[10,138] the overall incidence of congenital anomalies was nearly the same as the expected population incidence. The incidence of central nervous system malformations among IVF babies, however, was twice that expected.

Case-control studies examining the suspected association between ovulation induction and neural tube defects have produced mixed results. Cornel and colleagues[139,140] reported data from the Netherlands in which exposure to periconceptional clomiphene citrate was 3.2% among affected pregnancies and 0.8% among unaffected pregnancies (odds ratio [OR] 4.0; 95% CI, 1.0, 15.2). A similar study from Hungary[141] reported exposure to clomiphene citrate to be 0.4% among affected pregnancies and 0.1% among unaffected pregnancies (OR 5.8; 95% CI, 1.6, 20.4). Both studies identified cases from birth-defect registries, and both used population controls. Another case-control study from the United Kingdom[142] used a single hospital population as well as information from medical records recorded at the time of the first prenatal visit to examine the possible relationships between drug exposure and neural tube defects. Cases were matched by year of prenatal visit to two controls; four cases (3.7%) and five controls (2.3%) had been exposed to clomiphene citrate. An OR of 1.6 was reported (95% CI, 0.4, 6.2).

Vollset[143] performed a meta-analysis of these three case-control studies. The combined OR was estimated using the Mantel-Haenszel method[144] and reported as 2.9. The 95% CI was 1.3, 6.5. This indicated that the association between ovulation induction and neural tube defects was not due to chance.

Lastly, a population-based, case-control study from the United States[145] failed to find any increased risk for neural tube defects among women exposed to ovulation induction drugs during pregnancy. Five hundred seventy-one women who had a fetus or child with a neural tube defect were compared with 546 women who had a fetus or child with other abnormalities and 573 women who had an apparently normal fetus or child. Maternal interviews were used to collect information on exposure. The rate of maternal fertility-drug use was not significantly higher among cases compared with controls having other abnormalities (OR 1.3; 95% CI, 0.4, 4.5) or no abnormalities (OR 0.8; 95% CI, 0.6, 2.0).

Cancer
Inducing ovulation may be a risk factor for certain types of hormonally dependent cancers, particularly ovarian cancer. There

are two main etiological hypotheses. First, "incessant" ovulation may lead to malignant transformation.[146-148] Ovulation involves repeated disruption and minor mechanical trauma to the ovarian epithelium,[146,147,149] and in this process, the surface epithelium of the ovary may become entrapped to form an inclusion cyst.[149] Estrogen or estrogen precursors and gonadotropins then may be involved in the differentiation, proliferation, and eventual malignant transformation of the entrapped epithelium.[149] Second, persistent stimulation of the ovary by gonadotropins may have a direct carcinogenic effect or may act in conjunction with elevated concentrations of estrogens.[146,149,150] Excessive estrogen secretion has been implicated in ovarian, endometrial, and breast carcinoma,[151] and gonadotropin secretion has been implicated in ovarian cancer.[146,149] Estrogen also increases the frequency of mitotic activity, which may lead to malignant phenotypes.[146,149] These hypotheses are supported by evidence—albeit indirect—of a protective effect from factors that afford ovarian physiological rest periods (i.e., high parity, lactation, late menarche, early menopause, and oral contraceptive use).[146-148,152-158]

Data supporting concerns about a possible association between ovarian cancer and exposure to ovulation-induction drugs are accruing. There are several reported cases of ovarian cancer[159-162a] and breast cancer (two of which were bilateral)[163,164] following treatment with clomiphene citrate or hMG.

Few investigations directly evaluate the risks for cancer associated with ovulation induction. One study of cancer in a cohort of infertile women found no increase in cancer incidence associated with exposure to fertility drugs[165] A moderately increased risk of breast cancer in women having hormonal infertility was found, while women with other causes of infertility had excess risks of cancer of the ovary and thyroid. The authors concluded that infertile women treated with drugs to induce ovulation did not have a higher risk of cancer than did nontreated infertile women; rather, as other investigators showed,[166,167] hormonal infertility preceding treatment increased the risk of developing hormonal associated cancers. A recent collaborative analysis of 12 U.S. case-control studies refuted this conclusion when it was found that the risk of ovarian cancer among nulligravid women was 27 times higher if fertility drugs had been taken. At most, only a small fraction of excess risk was due to infertility per se.[167a]

Hydatidiform mole

Hydatidiform mole is a form of gestational, trophoblastic disease (a neoplasm of the trophoblast) that also includes invasive mole and choriocarcinoma.[168] Several investigators suggest that clomiphene citrate and hMG may be associated with the development of hydatidiform moles, but direct, causal relationships have not been established.[169] Epidemiological investigations have uncovered both genetic and environmental risk factors for the disease. Older women are at risk, which suggests that molar pregnancy could be a consequence of oocyte aging and pathological cell division of the fertilized oocyte.[168] On the other hand, abnormal cell division may result from exposure to ovulation-induction drugs.[170-173]

There are at least 16 reports of complete or partial hydatidiform mole following ovulation induction.[19,20,137,169,174-181] The disease, however, is rare, and most case series include too few observations to detect an increased incidence over that expected for the population in question.

CONCLUSIONS

Research has demonstrated that ovulation induction is associated with serious and sometimes life-threatening events. Severe ovarian hyperstimulation syndrome still occurs in approximately 1 in 50 to 1 in 100 women despite careful monitoring. Multiple pregnancy frequently complicates both induced and IVF pregnancies, and perinatal mortality is excessive. Recent data suggest that ovulation induction also may be a risk factor for extrauterine pregnancy, neural tube defects, defects in reproductive organogenesis, malignant neoplasms, and molar pregnancy.

Research implications

Well-designed epidemiological studies are urgently needed to ascertain the risks to women and their children associated with exposure to ovulation induction. Many of the suspected risks of ovulation induction are rare conditions that would be studied most appropriately with a retrospective, case-control design. These studies must account for the confounding effects of maternal age, preexisting health conditions (including infertility), reproductive history, family history, and other exposures. Some attempt also should be made to identify particularly sensitive organ systems, dose–response effects, and variation by length of time exposed to fertility drugs. Sample sizes must be adequate to detect significant differences.

Clinical implications

While many questions concerning the risks of ovulation induction still are unanswered, the weight of the evidence suggests that infertility problems should be managed conservatively. Until full appraisal of the risks of ovulation induction occurs, steps should be taken to limit the number of women exposed unnecessarily.

Care also must be taken not to treat subfertile women likely to conceive spontaneously in time. Treatment-independent pregnancy rates are proxy indicators of the extent of unnecessary treatment; studies of women accepted for IVF programs show that 7% to 28% conceive naturally either before receiving treatment or within 2 years after its discontinuation.[182–188] When women with bilateral tubal disease are excluded, treatment-independent pregnancy rates of 12% and 25% have been reported.[186,187] One clinic in Australia received notification that 450 spontaneous pregnancies had occurred in couples on a waiting list for IVF within a period of 5 years.[189]

Explicit clinical guidelines for infertility care should be developed. Several professional societies have attempted to do this,[190,191] and further refinement of their work (so that guidelines reflect the interests of health policy makers and the public at large) could do much to improve the standard of quality in infertility care. For example, guidelines could discourage clinics from imposing irrelevant and discriminatory social restrictions on admission to treatment (e.g., marital status and sexual preference) and encourage clinics to admit only those women who for biomedical reasons are appropriate candidates.

The number of stimulated cycles that women undergo also can be restricted. Prolonged exposure to ovulation-inducing agents may increase the risk of adverse physiological effects, but not the probability of conception. The effectiveness of ovulation induction when used alone decreases significantly after three cycles of treatment.[1,2] Likewise, the majority of women who conceive by IVF do so within three cycles of treatment.[192] Limiting the number of treatment cycles has the additional advantage of providing a clear end point to medical treatment so that alternative solutions can be sought.

Infertility counseling should be adequate and impartial. It must include full disclosure of the known and suspected risks of treatment and an accurate assessment of benefits. Social options such as adoption, foster parenting, and voluntary childlessness should be explored. It should not be assumed automatically that medical options are preferable.

Health policy implications

Health policy makers must address the growing concerns regarding the safety of the treatment of infertility. More effective drug-surveillance systems are needed as well. Currently, even countries requiring physicians to report all adverse effects of drugs to government agencies have not been able to overcome problems of underreporting. This seriously impedes the timely identification of short-term risks associated with drug exposure, and it makes no provision for assessing the long-term or intergenerational risks.

More effective quality-assurance systems are needed to protect the public. Until recently, most countries adopted a "hands-off" policy with regard to the regulation and monitoring of infertility treatment. Most countries have no capability for monitoring the outcomes of ovulation induction, no accreditation of infertility programs, and no special requirements for the training and certification of providers. Quality assurance should include the establishment of special registries for all women receiving ovulation-inducing drugs, record linkage with birth defects and cancer registries, mandatory reporting of all treatment outcomes, ongoing monitoring using selected indicators and independent audit, and enforceable sanctions for noncompliance.

REFERENCES

1. McEvoy GK, ed. American Hospital Formulary Services. Bethesda: American Society of Hospital Pharmacists, 1990:1443–1445.
2. United States Pharmacopeial Convention, Inc. Drug Information for the Health Care Professional. Rockville, MD: United States Pharmacopeial Convention, 1990:954–956, 1803–1805.
3. Shepard TH. Shepard's Catalog of Teratogenic Agents. Baltimore: Johns Hopkins University Press, 1990.
4. Trounson A. Preservation of human eggs and embryos. Fertil Steril 1986;46:1–12.
5. Wagner MG, St. Clair PA. Are in vitro fertilisation and embryo transfer of benefit to all? Lancet 1989;ii:1027–1030.
6. Scialli AR. The reproductive toxicity of ovulation induction. Fertil Steril 1986;45:315–323.
7. Diczfalusey E, Harlin J. Clinical-pharmacological studies on human menopausal gonadotropin. Human Reprod 1988;3:21–27.
8. MRC Working Party on Children Conceived of In Vitro Fertilisation. Births in Great Britain resulting from assisted conception, 1979–87. Br Med J 1990;300:1229–1233.
9. Medical Research Institute and Society of Assisted Reproductive Technology of the American Fertility Society. In vitro fertilization/embryo transfer in the United States: 1987 results from the National IVF/ET Registry. Fertil Steril 1989;51:14–18.
10. National Perinatal Statistics Unit and Fertility Society of Australia. IVF and GIFT Pregnancies: Australia and New Zealand, 1987. Sydney: National Perinatal Statistics Unit, 1988.
11. Hays PM, Smeltzer JS. Multiple gestation. Clin Obstet Gynecol 1986;29:264–285.
12. Botting BJ, MacDonald Davies I, MacFarlane AJ. Recent trends in the incidence of multiple births and associated mortality. Arch Dis Child 1987;62:941–950.
13. Hoffman EL, Bennett FC. Birth weight less than 800 grams: changing outcomes and influences of gender and gestation number. Pediatrics 1990;86:27–34.
14. Gemzell CA. Induction of ovulation with human gonadotropins. Rec Prog Hormonal Res 1965;21:179–204.
15. Whitelaw MJ. Clomiphene citrate: experience with 217 patients:

variation in response and unusual reactions. Fertil Steril 1966;17: 584–604.

16. Karow WG, Payne SA. Pregnancy after clomiphene citrate treatment. Fertil Steril 1968;19:351–362.

17. Van de Wiele RL, Turksoy RN. Treatment of amenorrhea and anovulation with human menopausal and chorionic gonadotropins. J Clin Endocrinol Metabol 1965;25:369–384.

18. Caspi E, Levin S, Bukovsky I, et al. Induction of pregnancy with human gonadotropins after clomiphene failure in menstruation ovulatory infertility patients. Isr J Med Sci 1974;10:249–255.

19. Ahlgren M, Kallen B, Rannevik G. Outcome of pregnancy after clomiphene therapy. Acta Obstet Gynecol Scand 1976;55:371–375.

20. MacGregor AH, Johnson JE, Bundi CA. Further clinical experience with clomiphene citrate. Fertil Steril 1968;19:616–622.

21. Hack M, Brish M, Serr DM, et al. Outcome of pregnancy after induced ovulation: follow-up of pregnancies and children born after clomiphene therapy. JAMA 1972;220:1329–1333.

22. Hack M, Brish M, Serr DM, et al. Outcome of pregnancy after induced ovulation: follow-up of pregnancies and children born after gonadotropin therapy. JAMA 1970:211:791–797.

23. Goldfarb AF, Morales A, Rakoff AE, et al. Critical review of 160 clomiphene-related pregnancies. Obstet Gynecol 1968;31:342–345.

24. Spadoni LR, Cox DW, Smith DC. Use of human menopausal gonadotropin for the induction of ovulation. Am J Obstet Gynecol 1974;120:988–993.

25. Oelsner G, Serr DM, Mashiak S, et al. The study of induction of ovulation with menotropins: analysis of results of 1897 treatment cycles. Fertil Steril 1978;30:538–544.

26. Tsapaulis AA, Zourlas PA, Comnino AC. Observations on 320 infertile patients treated with human gonadotropins (human menopausal gonadotropin/human chorionic gonadotropins). Fertil Steril 1978;29:492–495.

27. Gemzell CA. Experience with the induction of ovulation. J Reprod Med 1978;21(suppl):205–207.

28. Kistner RW. Induction of ovulation with clomiphene citrate (Clomid). South African J Obstet Gynecol 1967;5:25–35.

29. Adashi EY, Rock JA, Sapp KC, et al. Gestational outcome of clomiphene related conceptions. Fertil Steril 1979;31:620–626.

30. Butler JK. Clinical results with human gonadotrophins in anovulation using two alternative dosage schemes. Postgrad Med J 1972; 48:27–32.

31. Garcia JE, Jones GS, Wentz AC. The use of clomiphene citrate. Fertil Steril 1977;28:707–717.

32. Schwartz M, Jewelewicz R, Dyrenurth I, et al. The use of human menopausal and chorionic gonadotropins for induction of ovulation. Am J Obstet Gynecol 1974;138:801–807.

33. Murthy YS, Parekh MC, Arronet GH. Experience with clomiphene and cisclomiphene. Int J Fertil 1971;16:66–74.

34. U.S. Department of Health and Human Services. Proceedings of the International Collaborative Effort on Perinatal and Infant Mortality, Volumes I & II. Hyattsville, MD, 1988.

35. Schenker JG, Weinstein D. Ovarian hyperstimulation syndrome: a current survey. Fertil Steril 1978;30:255–268.

36. Polishuk W, Schenker JG. Ovarian overstimulation syndrome. Fertil Steril 1969;20:443–450.

37. Varma TR, Patel RH. Ovarian hyperstimulation syndrome: a case history and review. Acta Obstet Gynecol Scand 1988;67:579–584.

38. Zosmer A, Katz Z, Lancet M, et al. Adult respiratory distress syndrome complicating ovarian hyperstimulation syndrome. Fertil Steril 1987;47:524–526.

39. Rubessa S, Omodei V, Falsetti L, et al. Ovarian hyperstimulation syndrome (OHS): a case of severe OHS. Acta Eur Fertil 1989;20:15–17.

40. Magnus Ö, Tanbo T, Henriksen T, et al. Severe ovarian hyperstimulation syndrome. Case reports. Acta Eur Fertil 1988;19:89–92.

41. Gayrol MN, Millet D, Netter A. Syndrome d'hyperstimulation ovarienne. Commentaries sur la physiopathologic et le traitement, a propos de 3 observations (Ovarian hyperstimulation syndrome. Commentary on the pathophysiology and treatment of three cases). J Gynecol Obstet Biol Reprod 1975;4:255–266.

42. Engel T, Jewelewicz R, Dyrenfurth I, et al. Ovarian hyperstimulation syndrome. Report of a case with notes on pathogenesis and treatment. Am J Obstet Gynecol 1972;112:1052–1060.

43. Moneta E, Marana N, Garcea N, et al. Iatrogenic hyperstimulation of the ovaries with ascitis. Acta Eur Fertil 1977;8:155–166.

44. Neuwirth RS, Turksoy RN, Van de Wiele RL. Acute Meig's syndrome secondary to ovarian stimulation with human menopausal gonadotropins. Am J Obstet Gynecol 1965;91:977–981.

45. Lunenfeld B, Insler V. Classifications of amenorrheic states and their treatment by ovulation induction. Clin Endocrinol (Oxford) 1974;3:223–237.

46. Thompson C, Hansen M. Pergonal (menotropins): a summary of

clinical experience in induction of ovulation and pregnancy. Fertil Steril 1970;21:844–853.

47. Estebon-Alterriba J. Le syndrome d'hyperstimulation massive des ovaries (Massive ovarian hyperstimulation syndrome). Rev Fr Gynecol Obstet 1961;56:555–557.

48. Golan A, Ron-Ed R, Herman A, et al. Ovarian hyperstimulation following D-Trp-6 luteinizing hormone-releasing hormone microcapsules and menotropin for in vitro fertilization. Fertil Steril 1988;50:912–916.

49. Taymor ML. Gonadotropin therapy. JAMA 1968;203:362–364.

50. Roland M. Problems of ovulation induction with clomiphene citrate with report of a case of ovarian hyperstimulation. Obstet Gynecol 1970;35:55–62.

51. Chow KK, Choo HT. Ovarian hyperstimulation syndrome with clomiphene citrate. Case report. Br J Obstet Gynaecol 1984;91:1051–1052.

52. Southam AL, Janovski NA. Massive ovarian hyperstimulation with clomiphene citrate. JAMA 1962;181:443–445.

53. Scommegna A, Lash SR. Ovarian overstimulation, massive ascites and singleton pregnancy after clomiphene. JAMA 1969;207:753–755.

54. Rojanasakul A. Massive ascites following induction of ovulation with clomiphene citrate. J Med Assoc Thai 1988;71(suppl 2):86–88.

55. Germond M, Gaillard M-C, Senn A. Syndrome d'hyperstimulation ovarienne (Ovarian hyperstimulation syndrome). Arch Gynecol Obstet 1989;246:S53–64.

56. Mozes M, Bogokowsky H, Antebi E, et al. Thromboembolic phenomena after ovarian stimulation with human gonadotrophins. Lancet 1965;ii:1213–1215.

57. Hammerstein J. Dangers of overstimulation in use of clomiphene and gonadotropins. Geburtshilfe Fravenheilkd 1967;27:1125–1151.

58. Schenker JG, Polishuk WZ. Ovarian hyperstimulation syndrome. Obstet Gynecol 1975;46:23–28.

59. Kingsland CR, Collins JV, Rizk B, et al. Ovarian hyperstimulation presenting as acute hydrothorax after in vitro fertilization. Am J Obstet Gynecol 1989;161:381–382.

60. Corson SL, Batzer FR. Letter to the editor. Fertil Steril 1986;45:307–308.

61. Yovich JL, McColm SC, Turner SR, et al. Heterotopic pregnancy from in vitro fertilization. J In Vitro Fertil Embryo Transfer 1985;2:146–150.

62. Gemzell CA, Guillome J, Wang FC. Ectopic pregnancy following treatment with human gonadotropins. Am J Obstet Gynecol 1982;143:761–765.

63. Rein MS, Di Salvo DN, Friedman AJ. Heterotopic pregnancy associated with in vitro fertilization and embryo transfer: a possible role for routine vaginal ultrasound. Fertil Steril 1989;51:1057–1058.

64. Paldi E, Gergelz RZ, Abramovici H, et al. Clomiphene citrate induced simultaneous intra-extrauterine pregnancy: case report. Fertil Steril 1975;26:1140–1141.

65. Lower AM, Tyack AJ. Heterotopic pregnancy following in vitro fertilization and embryo transfer. Two case reports and a review of the literature. Hum Reprod 1989;4:726–728.

66. Bearman DM, Vieta PA, Snipes RD, et al. Heterotopic pregnancy after in vitro fertilization and embryo transfer. Fertil Steril 1986; 45:719–721.

67. Glassner MJ, Aron E, Eskin BA. Ovulation induction with clomiphene and rise in heterotopic pregnancies. A report of two cases. J Reprod Med 1990;35:175–178.

68. Laband SJ, Cherny WB, Finberg HS. Heterotopic pregnancy: report of four cases. Am J Obstet Gynecol 1988;158:437–438.

69. Dimitry ES, Oskarsson T, Mills M, et al. Combined intrauterine and cervical pregnancy from in vitro fertilization and embryo transfer. Fertil Steril 1989,52.871 875.

70. Berger MJ, Taymor ML. Simultaneous intrauterine and tubal pregnancies following ovulation induction. Am J Obstet Gynecol 1972; 113:812–813.

71. Raccuia JS, Neckles S, Butler D, et al. Synchronous intrauterine and ectopic pregnancy associated with clomiphene citrate. Surg Gynecol Obstet 1989;168:417–420.

72. Lund PR, Sielaff GW, Aiman EJ. In vitro fertilization patient presenting in hemorrhagic shock caused by unsuspected heterotopic pregnancy. Am J Emerg Med 1989;7:49–53.

73. Robertson S, Grant A. Combined intra-uterine and extra-uterine pregnancy in two patients treated with pituitary gonadotropins. Aust N Z J Obstet Gynecol 1972;12:253–254.

74. Gamberella FR, Marrs RP. Heterotopic pregnancy associated with assisted reproductive technology. Am J Obstet Gynecol 1989; 160:1520–1524.

75. Sondheimer SJ, Tureck RW, Blasco L, et al. Simultaneous ectopic pregnancy with intrauterine twin gestations after in vitro fertilization and embryo transfer. Fertil Steril 1985;43:313–316.

76. McLain PL, Kirkwood CR. Ovarian and intrauterine heterotopic pregnancy following clomiphene citrate ovulation induction. Report of a healthy live birth. J Fam Pract 1987;24:76–79.

77. Cope R. Two cases of combined intrauterine and extrauterine pregnancy. Radiology 1985;154:569–570.

78. Benacerraf RR, Rinehart JS, Schiff I. Sonographic diagnosis of simulataneous ectopic pregnancy. J Ultrasound Med 1985;4:331–332.

79. Koroly MV, Belsky DH. Heterotopic pregnancy as a result of induced ovulation. A report of two cases. J Reprod Med 1982;27:476–478.

80. Yovich JL, Stranger JD, Tuvik A, et al. Combined pregnancies following gonadotropin therapy. Am J Obstet Gynecol 1984;63:855–858.

81. Garcia JE. Letter to the editor. Fertil Steril 1989;52:874–875.

82. Bayati J, Garcia JE, Dorsey JA, et al. Combined intrauterine and cervical pregnancy from in vitro fertilization and embryo transfer. Fertil Steril 1989;51:725–727.

83. Porter R, Smith B, Ahuja K, et al. Combined twin ectopic gestation following in vitro fertilization and embryo transfer. J In Vitro Fertil Embryo Transfer 1986;3:330–332.

84. Oehninger S, Kreiner D, Bass MJ, et al. Abdominal pregnancy after in vitro fertilization and embryo transfer. Obstet Gynecol 1988;72:499–502.

85. Weyerman PC, Verhoeven AThM, Alberda ATh. Cervical pregnancy after in vitro fertilization and embryo transfer. Am J Obstet Gynecol 1989;161:1145–1146.

86. Falk RJ, Lackritz RM. Bilateral simultaneous tubal pregnancies after ovulation induction with clomiphene-menotropic combinations. Fertil Steril 1977;28:32–34.

87. Hann LE, Bachman DM, McArdle CR. Coexistent intrauterine and ectopic pregnancy: a reevaluation. Radiology 1984;152:151–154.

88. Reece EA, Petrie RH, Sirmans MF, et al. Combined intrauterine and extrauterine gestations: a review. Am J Obstet Gynecol 1983;146:323–330.

89. Richard SR, Stempel LE, Carlton BC. Heterotopic pregnancy: reappraisal of the incidence. Am J Obstet Gynecol 1982;142:928–930.

90. McBain JC, Evans JH, Pepperell RJ, et al. An unexpectedly high rate of ecotpic pregnancy following the induction of ovulation with human pituitary and chorionic gonadotropin. Br J Obstet Gynaecol 1980;87:5–9.

91. Kistner RW. Induction of ovulation with clomiphene citrate (Clomid). Obstet Gynecol Surv 1965;31:873–900.

92. Cohen J, Mayaux MJ, Guihard-Mascato-Guihard ML. Pregnancy outcomes after in vitro fertilization: a collaborative study on 2342 pregnancies. Ann N Y Acad Sci 1988;541:1–6.
93. Centers for Disease Control. Ectopic pregnancies—United States 1979–1980. MMWR 1984;33:201–202.
94. Marchbanks PA, Coulam CB, Annegers JF. An association between clomiphene citrate and ectopic pregnancy: a preliminary report. Fertil Steril 1985;44:268–270.
95. Folb PI, Dukes MNG. Drugs in Pregnancy. Amsterdam: Elsevier, 1990:285–298.
96. Bernstein HN. Some iatrogenic ocular diseases from systemically administered drugs. Int Ophthalmol Clin 1970;10:553–618.
97. Eneroth G, Forsberg V, Grant CA. Hydramnios and congenital cataracts induced in rats by clomiphene. Proc Eur Soc Study Drug Toxicity 1971;12:299–306.
98. Morris JM. Postcoital antifertility agents and their teratogenic effect. Contraception 1970;2:85–97.
99. Elbling L. Malformations induced by hormones in mice and their transmission to the offspring. Exp Pathol 1975;11:S115–122.
100. Elbling L. Does gonadotropin-induced ovulation in mice cause malformations in the offspring? Nature 1973;246:37–38.
101. Smith CM, Chrisman CL. Failure of exogenous gonadotropin controlled ovulation to cause digit abnormalities in mice. Nature 1975; 253:631–632.
102. Fujimoto S, Pahlavan N, Dukelow WR. Chromosomal abnormalities in rabbit preimplantation blastocysts induced by superovulation. J Reprod Fertil 1974;40:177–181.
103. Takagi N, Sasaki M. Digynic triploidy after superovulation in mice. Nature 1976;264:278–281.
104. Maudlin I, Fraser LR. The effect of PMSG dose on the incidence of chromosomal anomalies in mouse embryos fertilized in vitro. J Reprod Fertil 1977;50:275–280.
105. Elbling L, Colot M. Abnormal development and transport and increased sister-chromatid exchange in preimplantation embryos following superovulation in mice. Mutation Res 1987;147:189–195.
106. Elbling L, Colot M. Persistence of SCE-inducing damage in mouse embryos and fetuses following superovulation. Mutation Res 1987; 176:117–122.
107. Luckett DC, Mukherjee AB. Embryonic characteristics in superovulated mouse strains. J Heredity 1987;77:39–42.
108. Kaufman MH. Analysis of the first cleavage division to determine

the sex ratio and incidence of chromosome anomalies at conception in the mouse. J Reprod Fertil 1973;35:67–72.

109. Vickers AD. Delayed fertilization and chromosomal anomalies in mouse embryos. J Reprod Fertil 1969;20:69–76.

110. Gorwill RH, Steele HD, Saida IR. Heterotopic columnar epithelium and adenosis in the vagina of the mouse after neonatal treatment with clomiphene citrate. Am J Obstet Gynecol 1982;144:529–532.

111. Clark JH, McCormack SA. The effect of clomid and other triphenylethylene derivatives during pregnancy and the neonatal period. J Steroid Biochem 1980;12:47–53.

112. Clark JH, McCormack SA. Clomid or nafoxidine administered to neonatal rats causes reproductive tract abnormalities. Science 1977; 197:164–165.

113. McCormack SA, Clark JH. Clomid administration to pregnant rats causes abnormalities of the reproductive tract in offspring and mothers. Science 1979;204:629–631.

114. Clark JH, Guthrie SC. The estrogenic effects of clomiphene during the neonatal period in the rat. J Steroid Biochem 1983;18:513–517.

115. Gorwill RH, Steele HD, Sarda IR. The effect of clomiphene citrate on the developing mouse vagina. Fertil Steril 1980;34:190.

116. Branham WS, Zehr DR, Chen JJ, et al. Uterine abnormalities in rats exposed neonatally to diethystilbestrol, ethynylestrodrol, or clomiphene citrate. Toxicology 1988;51:201–212.

117. Branham WS, Zehr DR, Chen JJ, et al. Alterations in developing rat uterine populations after neonatal exposure to estrogens and antiestrogens. Teratol 1988;38:271–279.

118. Cunha GR, Taguchi O, Namikawa R, et al. Teratogenic effects of clomiphene, tamoxifen and diethylstilbestrol on the developing human female genital tract. Hum Pathol 1987;18:1132–1143.

119. Boué JG, Boué A. Increased frequency of chromosomal anomalies in abortions after induced ovulation. Lancet 1973;i:679–680.

120. Boué J, Boué A, Lazar P. Retrospective and prospective epidemiological studies of 1500 karyotyped spontaneous human abortions. Teratology 1973;12:11–26.

121. Sandler B. Anencephaly and ovulation stimulation. Lancet 1973; ii:379.

122. Field B, Kerr C. Ovulation stimulation and defects of neural tube closure. Lancet 1974;ii:1511.

123. Barrett C, Hakim C. Anencephaly, ovulation stimulation, subfertility and illegitimacy. Lancet 1973;ii:916–917.

124. Dyson JL, Kohler HG. Anencephaly and ovulation stimulation. Lancet 1973;i:1256–1257.

125. Biale Y, Lenenthal H, Altaras M, et al. Anencephaly and clomiphene-induced pregnancy. Acta Obstet Gynecol Scand 1978;57: 483–484.
126. Singhi M, Singhi S. Possible relationship between clomiphene and neural tube defects. J Pediatr 1978;93:152.
127. Laing IA, Steer CR, Dudgeon J, et al. Clomiphene and congenital retinopathy. Lancet 1981;ii:1107.
128. Ford WDA, Little KET. Fetal ovarian dysplasia possibly associated with clomiphene. Lancet 1981;ii:1107.
129. Melamed I, Birjanover Y, Hammer J, et al. Hepatoblastoma in an infant born to a mother after hormonal treatment for infertility. N Engl J Med 1982;307:820.
130. Harlap S. Ovulation induction and congenital malformations. Lancet 1976;ii:961.
131. Berman P. Congenital abnormalities associated with maternal clomiphene ingestion. Lancet 1975;ii:878.
132. Ylikorkala O. Congenital anomalies and clomiphene. Lancet 1975; ii:1262–1263.
133. Oakley GP, Flynt JW. Increased prevalence of Down's syndrome (Mongolism) among the offspring of women treated with ovulation inducing agents. Teratology 1972;5:264.
134. Batres GM, Collado R, Moro S, et al. Tetralogy of Fallot in a blastocystic implantation. Am J Cardiol 1987;59:1206.
135. Marino B, Marcelletti C. Complex congenital heart disease after in vitro fertilization. Am J Dis Child 1989;143:1136–1137.
136. Newberne JW, Kuhn WL, Elsea JR. Toxicologic studies on clomiphene. Toxicol Applied Pharmacol 1966;9:44–56.
137. Kurachi K, Aono T, Minagawa J, et al. Congenital malformations of newborn infants after clomiphene induced ovulation. Fertil Steril 1983;40:187–189.
138. Lancaster PAL. Congenital malformations after in-vitro fertilisation. Lancet 1987;ii:1392–1393.
139. Cornel MC, TenKate LP, Te Murman CJ. Ovulation induction, in vitro fertilisation and neural tube defects. Lancet 1989;ii:1530.
140. Cornel MD, TenKate LP, Dukes MNG, et al. Ovulation induction and neural tube defects. Lancet 1989;i:1386.
141. Czeizel A. Ovulation induction and neural tube defects. Lancet 1989;ii:167.
142. Cuckle H, Wald N. Ovulation induction and neural tube defects. Lancet 1989;ii:1281.
143. Vollset SE. Ovulation induction and neural tube defects. Lancet 1990;i:178.

144. Mantel N, Haenzel W. Statistical aspects of the analysis of data from retrospective studies of disease. J Natl Cancer Inst 1959;22:719–748.

145. Mills JL, Simpson JL, Rhoads GG, et al. Risk of neural tube defects in relation to maternal fertility and fertility drug use. Lancet 1990; ii:103–104.

146. Fishel S, Jackson P. Follicle stimulation for high tech pregnancies: are we playing it safe? Br Med J 1989;299:309–311.

147. Fathalla MF. Incessant ovulation—a factor in ovarian neoplasia? Lancet 1971;ii:163.

148. Cassagrande JF, Louie EW, Pike MC, et al. Incessant ovulation and ovarian cancer. Lancet 1979;ii:170–172.

149. Cramer DW, Welch WR. Determinants of ovarian cancer risk II. Inferences regarding pathogenesis. J Natl Cancer Inst 1983;71:717–721.

150. Stadel BV. The etiology of ovarian cancer. Am J Obstet Gynecol 1975;123:772–780.

151. Henderson BF, Ross R, Bernstein L. Estrogens as a cause of human cancer: the Richard and Helda Rosenthal Foundation Award Lecture. Cancer Res 1988;48:246–253.

152. Joly DJ, Lilienfeld AM, Diamond EL, et al. An epidemiologic study of the relationship of reproductive experience to cancer of the ovary. Am J Epidemiol 1974;99:190–209.

153. Hildreth NG, Kelsey JL, Li Volsi, et al. An epidemiologic study of epithelial carcinoma of the ovary. Am J Epidemiol 1981;114:398–405.

154. Risch HA, Weiss NS, Lyon JL. Events of reproductive life and the incidence of epithelial ovarian cancer. Am J Epidemiol 1983;117:128–139.

155. Beral V, Fraser P, Chilvers C. Does pregnancy protect against ovarian cancer? Lancet 1978;i:1083–1087.

156. Nasca PC, Greenwald P, Chowst S. An epidemiologic case-control study of ovarian cancer and reproductive factors. Am J Epidemiol 1984;119:705–713.

157. Cramer DW, Hutchinson GB, Welch WR. Determinants of ovarian cancer risk I. Reproductive experience and family history. J Natl Cancer Inst 1983;4:711–716.

158. LaVecchia C, Franceschi S, Decarli A, et al. Risk factors for endometrial cancer at different ages. J Natl Cancer Inst 1984;3:667–671.

159. Bamford PN, Steele SJ. Uterine and ovarian carcinoma in a patient receiving gonadotropin therapy. Case report. Br J Obstet Gynaecol 1982;89:962–964.

160. Ben-Hur H, Dgani R, Lancet M, et al. Ovarian carcinoma masquerading as ovarian hyperstimulation syndrome. Acta Obstet Gynecol Scand 1986;65:813–814.

161. Carter ME, Joyce DN. Ovarian carcinoma in a patient hyperstimulated by gonadotropin therapy for in vitro fertilization: a case report. J In Vitro Fertil Embryo Transfer 1987;4:126–128.

162. Atlas M, Menczer J. Massive hyperstimulation and borderline carcinoma of the ovary. Acta Obstet Gynecol Scand 1982;61:261–263.

162a. Kulkarni R, McGarry JM. Follicular stimulation and ovarian cancer. Br Med J 1989;299:740.

163. Bolton PM. Bilateral breast cancer associated with clomiphene. Lancet 1977;ii:1176.

164. Laing RW, Glaser MG, Barrett GS. A case of breast carcinoma in association with in vitro fertilization. J Roy Soc Med 1989;82:503.

165. Ron E, Lunenfeld B, Menczer J, et al. Cancer incidence in a cohort of infertile women. Am J Epidemiol 1987;125:780–790.

166. Brindon LA, Melton LJ III, Malkasian GD Jr., et al. Cancer risk after evaluation for infertility. Am J Epidemiol 1989;129:712–722.

167. Cowan LD, Gordis L, Tonascia JA. Breast cancer incidence in women with a history of progesterone deficiency. Am J Epidemiol 1981;114:209–217.

167a. Whitlemore AS, Harris R, Hayne J, et al. Characteristics relating to ovarian cancer risk: collaborative analysis of 12 U.S. case-control studies. Am J Epidemiol 1992;10:1184–1203.

168. Craighill MC, Cramer DW. Epidemiology of complete molar pregnancy. J Reprod Med 1984;29:784–787.

169. Weiss DB, Aboulafia Y. Ectopic gestation and hydatidiform mole in clomiphene-induced pregnancies. Lancet 1975;ii:1094–1095.

170. Yoshimura Y, Hosoi Y, Atlas SJ, et al. Effect of clomiphene citrate on in vitro ovulated ova. Fertil Steril 1986;45:800–804.

171. Laufer N, Reich R, Braw R, et al. Effect of clomiphene citrate on preovulatory rat follicles in culture. Biol Reprod 1982;27:463–471.

172. Schmidt GE, Kim MH, Mansour R, et al. The effects of clomiphene and zuclomiphene citrates on mouse embryos fertilized in vitro and in vivo. Am J Obstet Gynecol 1986;154:727–736.

173. Baufer N, Pratt BM, DeCherney AH, et al. The in vivo and in vitro effects of clomiphene citrate on ovulation, fertilization and development of cultured mouse oocytes. Am J Obstet Gynecol 1983;147:633–639.

174. Portuondo JA, Camarero MC, Matra JC, et al. Hydatidiform mole following successful gonadotropin ovulation induction and donor artificial insemination. Int J Gynecol Obstet 1982;20:207–209.

175. Miles PA, Taylor HB, Hill WC. Hydatidiform mole in a clomiphene-related pregnancy: a case report. Obstet Gynecol 1971;37:358–359.
176. Erving HW, Bower JE. Hydatidiform mole following clomiphene therapy. Int Surg 1967;47:493–496.
177. Wajntraub G, Kamar R, Pardo Y. Hydatidiform mole after treatment with clomiphene. Fertil Steril 1974;25:904–905.
178. Mor-Joseph S, Anteby SO, Granat M, et al. Recurrent molar pregnancies associated with clomiphene citrate and human gonadotropins. Am J Obstet Gynecol 1985;151:1085–1086.
179. Schneiderman CI, Waxman B. Clomid therapy and subsequent hydatidiform mole formation. Obstet Gynecol 1972;39:787–788.
180. Zbella EA, Vermesh M, Depp G, et al. Coexistent complete hydatidiform mole and fetus after therapy with human menopausal gonadotropin. A case report. J Reprod Med 1984;29:760–762.
181. Ohmichi M, Tasaka K, Suchara N, et al. Hydatidiform mole in a triplet pregnancy following gonatropin therapy. Acta Obstet Gynecol Scand 1986;65:523–524.
182. Jarrell J, Gwatkin R, Lumsden B, et al. An in vitro fertilization and embryo transfer pilot study: treatment-dependent and treatment-independent pregnancies. Am J Obstet Gynecol 1986;154:231–235.
183. Haney AF, Hughes CL Jr, Whitesides DB, et al. Treatment-independent, treatment-associated and pregnancies after additional therapy in a program of in vitro fertilization and embryo transfer. Fertil Steril 1987;47:634–638.
184. Damewood MD, Rock JA. Treatment independent pregnancy with operative laparoscopy for endometriosis in an in vitro fertilization program. Fertil Steril 1988;50:463–465.
185. Correy JF, Watkins RA, Bradfield GF, et al. Spontaneous pregnancies and pregnancies as a result of treatment in an in vitro fertilization program terminating in ectopic pregnancies or spontaneous abortions. Fertil Steril 1988;50:85–88.
186. Ben-Rafael Z, Mashiach S, Dor J, et al. Treatment independent pregnancy after in vitro fertilization and embryo transfer trial. Fertil Steril 1986;45:564–567.
187. Roh SI, Awadalla SG, Friedman CI, et al. In vitro fertilization and embryo transfer: treatment-dependent versus independent pregnancies. Fertil Steril 1987;48:982–986.
188. Collins JA, Wrixin W, Janes LB, et al. Treatment-independent pregnancy among infertilie couples. N Engl J Med 1983;309:1201–1206.
189. Saunders DM, Mathews M, Lancaster PAL. The Australian Register: current research and future role. Ann N Y Acad Sci 1988;541:7–21.

190. European Society of Human Reproduction and Embryology. Safety and Standards Committee. Recommendations for in vitro fertilization and embryo transfer. ESHRE News Lett 1990;10:9–14.
191. American Fertility Society. Minimal standards for programs of in vitro fertilization. Fertil Steril 1986;46:87S–88S.
192. Page H. Calculating the effectiveness of in vitro fertilization. A review. Br J Obstet Gynaecol 1989;96:334–339.

8

Physiological and Psychosocial Risks of the New Reproductive Technologies
■

LENE KOCH

In vitro fertilization, GIFT, and related technologies have become widely available without adequate assessment of their risks. Most research has focused on possible short-term risks to the fetus or infant. The risks for women, however, the true patients in IVF and GIFT, seldom have been considered.

Not all risks are physiological. Involuntary childlessness very often is a psychologically stressful condition, and both IVF and GIFT very often contribute to those stresses. Therefore, the impact of both the condition and the treatment must be considered.

Also, risks are not related exclusively to the individual. The health and psychosocial effects of both infertility and its treatment have political and social ramifications for individuals, families, and society.

This chapter reviews what is known about the health risks of specific IVF and GIFT procedures as well as the psychosocial effects of such treatment. The risks for women and their children associated with ovulation induction are discussed elsewhere.

PHYSICAL AND PSYCHOSOCIAL RISKS ASSOCIATED WITH TREATMENT

Complications of oocyte retrieval

Several complications can arise from retrieving oocytes. The most common methods of oocyte retrieval are laparoscopy and ultrasonically guided puncture. Laparoscopy, the older method, is a surgical technique that requires anesthesia and distension of the abdomen with carbon-dioxide gas. While infrequent, anesthesia accidents may lead to serious morbidity and even death;[1] additional rare complications of laparoscopy include misplacement of carbon dioxide, causing acidosis and cardiac arrest; air embolism; stress hormone response; puncture of internal organs; hemorrhage; and resurgence of both PID and pelvic adhesions.[1]

Ultrasonically directed oocyte retrieval is now replacing laparoscopy. This method is safer and less expensive as it avoids the need for both general anesthesia and hospitalization. In the transabdominal method, a catheter is inserted through the abdomen and the full urinary bladder to reach the ovary, while the transducer is placed on the abdomen. In the transvaginal method, the ultrasound transducer and the catheter are inserted in the vagina, thus getting closer to the ovary than by the transabdominal approach. The transvaginal method also is preferred because it is less painful.

Either technique carries a risk of infection, urinary disturbance, and visceral injury,[2] and visceral injury as well as ovarian trauma followed by bleeding leads to intrapelvic adhesions.[2] In turn, intrapelvic adhesions can exacerbate preexisting infertility or cause infertility in normal women seeking treatment for male factors. Two Israeli clinics reported such cases in 1987,[3] and physicians from the Sherman Institute of Fertility[3] commented:

> It is a well documented fact that ovarian surgery . . . predisposes the patient to the development of multiple adhesions in the pelvis. In fact any surgical procedure involving the accumulation of blood-stained fluid in the intraperitoneal space involves the formation of postoperative adhesions. . . . Other predisposing factors for the formation of adhesions, however,

such as tissue trauma or manipulation resulting in tissue reaction or puncture of the ovaries or flushing of the follicular bed with medium added with heparin, obviously cannot be avoided during ovum pick-up.

Oocyte retrieval therefore must be considered a possible cause of mechanical infertility. The frequency of complications according to one Scandinavian survey ($n = 6,350$ embryo transfers) is 0.5% ($n = 318$ embryo transfers).[4]

Complications of embryo or egg transfer

Women undergoing IVF or GIFT also are at risk for infection from embryo or egg transfer. Bacteria or viruses may be introduced by contaminated equipment, contaminated cell-culture media, or through sperm, donor sperm, and donor eggs. For example, hundreds of women in the Netherlands were exposed to hepatitis B through contaminated culture medium in 1987 and 1988.[5] In this case, the supplier of the blood product used in the culture medium as well as the clinics involved failed to establish who would take responsibility for testing the blood product.

The process of embryo or egg transfer also may increase the risk of ectopic pregnancy. Most population-based studies show that 5% to 7% of all IVF and GIFT pregnancies implant outside the uterus.[6,7] The expected frequency of ectopic pregnancy is approximately 1%.[8] Ectopic pregnancies always result in a dead fetus, and they may be dangerous—even life-threatening—to the woman. Ectopic pregnancy also can exacerbate infertility.

The incidence of multiple births is increasing among the general population, largely as a result of treatment for infertility.[9,10] A recent study in the United Kingdom demonstrated that from 1980 to 1985 more than one-third of all mothers of triplets and nearly three-quarters of all mothers of quadruplets had taken fertility drugs. Since 1985, much of the increase in the rate of multiple births has been caused by IVF, GIFT, and associated procedures.[9,11]

Multiple births occur in one out of four IVF and GIFT pregnancies.[6,7] Multiple births increase the risk of spontanous abortion, pregnancy-induced hypertension, early labor, and placental dysfunction,[10] and the practice of transferring more than one embryo or egg per treatment cycle is directly related to the incidence of multiple birth.[12] Clinicians have found that IVF and GIFT success rates depend on the number of embryos or eggs transferred.[12] The greater the number of embryos or eggs transferred, however, the higher the risk of multiple births.[12] Despite the risk, transferring three or more embryos or eggs per treatment cycle is still a common practice.[6,7]

Twins and higher-order multiple births frequently are of low birth weight.[10] In the U.K. study, more than half the quadruplets and over a quarter of the triplets weighed less than 1500 g at birth, and some died in the neonatal period. Twenty-eight percent of all live-born triplets and 62% of live-born quadruplets spent 1 month or more in the intensive care unit as well.[9,11] Despite improvements in neonatal intensive care, preterm birth and low birth weight remain important causes of infant death and long-term physical handicap, mental retardation, and hearing and vision impairment.

Having a critically ill child in an intensive care unit is an extremely stressful experience. In countries such as the United States, where no national health insurance system exists, the financial burden alone can overwhelm a family. This only adds to the fact that losing a much-wanted child is a terrible tragedy that is not diminished even if another child survives.

Multiple births likely will create many psychosocial problems for those responsible for the care and welfare of these children. In a study of 20 sets of triplets, Syrop and Varner[13] found that 3 sets required placement in foster homes. When three, four, or five children survive the perinatal period, it is likely that the care they will require places such extraordinary demands on their parents that they cannot cope alone for any length of time.[10] Families may need to either move their home or build additional rooms onto existing structures.[9] Ordinary domestic life must be organized with military precision as well.[9] Having a child, or several children, with physical or mental handicaps or both poses additional problems for families; these children may require special schooling, appliances, and attention from both their parents and teachers.

Selective reduction of excess fetuses has been presented as a solution to the problem of multiple pregnancies. This invasive and ethically dubious procedure should be considered yet another risk to women undergoing IVF or GIFT. Different techniques may be used to destroy excess fetuses depending on the preference of the doctor and the gestational age of the pregnancy. The fetal sac may be injected with potassium chloride, or the fetus may be exsanguinated or aspirated.

The legality of this procedure may rely on an interpretation of abortion law.[14] It has been claimed as legal because the pregnancy as such is not terminated.[14] Abortion generally is thought of as a procedure for the termination of unwanted or damaged pregnancies; therefore, the idea that a wanted and perhaps normal fetus would be aborted does not sit well with many ethicists. The long-term consequences of fetal reduction are unknown.

Birth complications

In vitro fertilization and GIFT pregnancies are more often delivered by cesarean section. A recent Australian survey reported the incidence of cesarean section among IVF and GIFT pregnancies to be 46.7% in 1987, which is three times higher than that expected for the general population.[6] A Dutch multicenter survey reported a cesarean section rate of 31% among IVF and GIFT births.[15]

Some argue that the risk of cesarean section is related to the increased anxiety that naturally follows when such extraordinary efforts and expense are involved in achieving a pregnancy. The current rhetoric holds that no particular reason exists to treat an IVF or GIFT pregnancy and birth as high risk. One Swedish study, however, showed that of 44 IVF and GIFT cesarean sections, only 7 were performed for psychological indications.[16]

Psychosocial impact of infertility treatment

In vitro fertilization and GIFT treatment do not resolve the problem of infertility for the majority of treated patients, and treatment failure may produce feelings of grief, anxiety, and depression. Greenfield and coworkers[17] described three cases of depression following IVF or GIFT failure, and they compared the reaction to a grief reaction. Baram and colleagues[18] reported a depressive reaction in 66% of women and 44% of men after a failed IVF or GIFT cycle. Also, both Leiblum and colleagues[19] as well as Reading and coworkers[20] compared women before and after IVF or GIFT treatment and found significantly higher depression scores after failed treatment cycles.

Such grief or depression responses may be influenced by the degree of investment in the idea of pregnancy. Women undergoing IVF or GIFT may become hopeful for and invested in the notion of successfully establishing a pregnancy as they proceed through the highly visible procedures involved in their treatment.[21] They may see ultrasonographic pictures of follicle development and receive overly optimistic information on their hormone levels. They will be informed of the success or failure of their eggs to fertilize as well as the development of the resulting embryos. As a result, they may develop unrealistic beliefs regarding success.[21,22] Women also may be given either incomplete or inaccurate information concerning their chances of achieving a live birth with IVF or GIFT,[23] which further increases their risk for depressive reactions and feelings of loss.

Several studies have described the so-called "roller-coaster effect"—the emotional peaks and troughs experienced in the time between one step of an IVF treatment and the next.[24] There may be great happiness felt at being included in a program, followed by distress at having to wait for treatment, followed by happiness to have eggs extracted and successfully fertilized, and then distress again when the eggs did not implant. This roller-coaster effect may be expected to repeat itself during every IVF cycle the woman undergoes.

Recent studies also have shown that once a woman embarks on IVF or GIFT, it is very hard to decide to stop.[21–23] Similarly, some years after failed treatment, women may feel emotional distress and an inability to come to grips with their infertility.[21] The new reproductive technologies may have made a woman's adjustment to infertility more difficult.[21] The hope now always exists that a new treatment "breakthrough" will become available, and it also can be difficult now to discount the possibility that one last try might bring success.[21] For example, Leiblum and coworkers[19] found that 90% of women assessed at least 8 months after completing IVF or GIFT treatment said they would resume the process if a new treatment became available. The hope for a new and a better treatment may cause women to delay seeking alternative solutions, such as adoption, until they have passed the eligible age.

Another phenomemon, known as "insecure motherhood," also is a risk of IVF and GIFT.[25–27] Insecure motherhood results from the confusion of traditional, culturally established notions of familial relationships brought about by the separation of the social from the genetic and physiological aspects of motherhood. This is quite obvious when egg donation is involved, but it seems the mere possibility that gametes may be confused in the laboratory has led to fear that doctors will make a mistake and use sperm from a man other than the woman's partner, or even another woman's eggs. Others fear that experiments will occur on their excess embryos; in one study, this was reported to be one of the most stressful aspects of treatment.[28]

LONG-TERM RISKS FOR CHILDREN, FAMILIES, AND SOCIETY

Publicly financed IVF and GIFT are not open to all. For some women and their families, the economic burden of treatment is overwhelming. Likewise, the costs borne by society and its health care system also are quite high (see Chapter 5 of this volume) and thus may inadvertently siphon off resources from other health and social services.

Few studies exist on the development of children after IVF or GIFT. Few include control groups, and results are mixed. Yovich and colleagues[29] studied a small sample of 20 children at the age of 12 months. Six of these children suffered respiratory problems in the neonatal period, but only 1 child was below the expected developmental level. Mushin and coworkers[30] studied 33 children between 12 and 37 months of age, and 4 had major physical or psychological problems. Seven had minor problems. Also, Morin and colleagues[31] matched 83 IVF and GIFT children with 105 control children and assessed them at 12 to 30 months of age. No significant differences in the rate of physical or neurological abnormalities or psychological development were found. To date, however, no study has had an adequate sample size, methodology, or long-enough follow-up to determine what indeed the risks are. In developmental testing, any assessment done before the age of 18 months (when language skills should have developed in most children) is inconclusive.

Adjunct procedures such as embryo or egg freezing, gamete donation, zona drilling, and related procedures lead to other questions concerning the risks and benefits of treatment for families, children, and society. No one knows the long-term physiological or psychological impact on the children of such procedures, and no one knows the long-term impact on society of treating gametes, embryos, and ultimately children, as commodities.

CONCLUSIONS

Significant physical risks are associated with IVF and GIFT procedures, and psychosocial risks are involved both with treatment failure and success. All too often, however, attempts at openly discussing these risks are hampered by emotional appeals for the plight of the infertile, or even dismissed with the argument that the potential benefits of these technologies to the infertile outweigh their attendant risks.

Does this argument have any merit? What, indeed, is it like to be unable to bear children? Reading and Kerin[21] described the experience of infertility as

> a major life event involving stress and a sense of impending loss. There is a feeling of being out of control of one's body. That may lead infertile people to selectively encode cues related to inadequacy, lack of femininity, information about

prospects of pregnancy and the stigma of not being able to conceive. Infertility may also trigger past associations with loss or failure. Such associations may include the loss of a parent or a past pregnancy, through either spontaneous or elective abortion. Infertility may also trigger a search for further confirmatory experiences of inadequacy, such as looking for signs of inadequacy as wife or homemaker and thus sabotaging a marital relationship. The attendant guilt and self-blame may amplify this process.

Traditional psychodynamic theories have likened infertility to a loss experience, and so they have drawn on the stages of grieving to describe the emotions of infertile women and men.[21] Women (and men) may experience feelings of loss for the "imagined child." Infertility also may threaten one's self-concept as well as one's ability to adopt certain social roles and to fulfill certain adult role expectations.[21,32] Because of the social importance attached to pregnancy, childbearing, and parenting, infertility can become a symbol of role failure for some.[21,32] Spouses may feel they have disappointed each other and their parents, and they may be given subtle or not-so-subtle messages that either they are not trying hard enough or they will never feel "complete" without a child.[33,34] Thus, the experience of infertility itself, whether treated or not with IVF or GIFT, may have a negative or distruptive impact on people's lives.

It should be pointed out, however, that most (if not all) research to date on the psychosocial impact of infertility and involuntary childlessness has focused on the experiences and accounts of either clinic or former clinic patients. Results of studies on such patients may be biased by two conditions: clinic patients are not representative of all infertile people, and clinic patients may "pick up" the opinions and attitudes of care providers and researchers who fervently believe that infertility is both a tragedy and a crisis. Therefore, the studies reviewed herein may give an incomplete or distorted view of the experience of infertility.

Perhaps an entirely different set of attitudes and experiences would be found in those who opted not to receive IVF or GIFT treatment and who instead chose other medical treatments, adoption, or childlessness. After all, a wealth of research on the subject of psychosocial aspects of chronic disease demonstrates that people are capable, most of the time, of both adapting to and coping with everything from cancer surgery to long-term mental illness. It is hard to believe that the experience of infertility is any different; indeed, it is prejudicial to approach a study of infertility's psychosocial aspects assuming that infertility is an unrelenting source of misery and pain.

From a clinical perspective, these data strongly indicate that women and their partners should have the opportunity to receive counseling both before and after IVF or GIFT treatment. Some provision must be made for long-term support as well; if IVF is not successful, then the grieving process may continue for some time. IVF and GIFT clinicians must be able to handle that grief and depressive reactions in their clients, because they likely will be first to recognize these signs. This may require additional training, and it certainly requires the establishment of close ties with psychologists and social workers.

The technology for both IVF and GIFT as well as adjunct technologies such as zona drilling, embryo freezing, and gamete donation have not been accompanied by careful scrutiny and analysis of the risks involved. Indeed, even when risks are clearly established (as with multiple pregnancy), there has been no discernable attempt to reduce these risks by altering procedures and protocols. There also has been an appalling lack of follow-up studies to determine the long-term health, psychological, and social consequences of these procedures.

Furthermore, characteristics of the mother such as advanced reproductive age or underlying infertility all too often are used to explain the higher-than-expected risks of ectopic pregnancy, spontaneous abortion, cesarean section, and so forth. While maternal characteristics may indeed be the true underlying "cause" of some complications in some cases, the complications never would have occurred had the woman not been subjected to treatment. Regardless of the cause, the end result is the same: it is folly to isolate the technology from its application. For a discussion of IVF and GIFT in the broader context of infertility care, it is necessary to discuss the technology not as a theoretical abstraction but as it actually is practiced in the clinic.

To minimize the risks, some clinics have established patient-selection criteria that exclude women at highest risk (e.g., women over 40 years of age) and those who may not be psychologically suitable.[35] It must be remembered, however, that IVF, GIFT, and related technologies were marketed in many countries by the medical community and accepted by health authorities only as a last-resort treatment for infertile women who had tried everything else or for whom no medical alternative existed. Today, these technologies have become the treatment of choice for infertility caused by everything from tubal blockage to male factors.

Therefore, when an infertile couple considers IVF or GIFT, or when health policy makers consider how best to spend limited health care resources, the known risks of this technology must be accepted or rejected per se. They must not be minimized by referring to possible future modification of the method or with stirring emotional pleas, nor is it appropriate to accept the elevated incidence of serious complications on the basis of rationalizing the underlying etiology.

REFERENCES

1. Holmes HB. In vitro fertilization: reflections on the state of the art. Birth 1988;15:134–144.
2. Ashkenazi J, Ben David M, Feldberg D, et al. Abdominal complications following ultrasonically guided percutaneous transvesical collection of oocytes for in vitro fertilization. J In Vitro Fertil Embryo Transfer 1987;4:316–318.
3. Ashkenazi J, Feldberg D, Ben David M, et al. Ovum pickup for in vitro fertilization. A cause of mechanical infertility. J In Vitro Fertil Embryo Transfer 1987;4:242–245.
4. Bergh TH. Vilka är de medicinska riskerne for paret? (What are the medical risks for the couple?) Assisterad befruktning vid ofrivillig barnlöshet. Konsensuskonferens 24–26 April, SPRI, Stockholm, 1990:69.

5. Holmes HB. Hepatitis—yet another risk of in vitro fertilization. Reprod Genet Eng 1989;2:29–37.
6. National Perinatal Statistics Unit, Fertility Society of Australia. IVF and GIFT Pregnancies, Australia and New Zealand 1987. Sydney: National Perinatal Statistics Unit, 1988.
7. Medical Research Institute and Society of Assisted Reproductive Technology of the American Fertility Society. In Vitro Fertilization/ Embryo Transfer in the United States: 1987. Results from the National IVF/ET Registry. Fertil Steril 1989;51:14–18.
8. Centers for Disease Control. Ectopic Pregnancy—United States, 1979–1980. MMWR 1984;33:201–202.
9. Price F. Too much of a good thing. New Scientist 1990;18:29–30.
10. Price FV. The risk of high multiparity with IVF/ET. Birth 1988; 15:157–163.
11. Three, Four or More—a Study of Triplet and Higher Order Births. London: Her Majesty's Stationery Office, 1990.
12. Lancaster P. How many oocytes/embryos should be transplanted? Lancet 1987;ii:273.
13. Syrop CH, Varner MW. Triplet gestation: maternal and neonatal implications. Acta Genet Med Gemellol 1985;34:81–88.
14. Brahams D. Assisted reproduction and selective reduction of pregnancy. Lancet 1987;ii:1409–1410.
15. Haan G, Van Steen R, Rutten F. Evaluatie van in-vitro-fertilisatie (Evaluation of in vitro fertilization). Vakgroep Ekonomie van de Gezondheidsorg. Thesis, Rijsuniversiteit Limburg, Maastricht, 1989:60–62.
16. Wennerholm U-B. Hur forloper graviditet och forlossning for mor och foster? (What happens during pregnancy and birth for mother and fetus?) Assisterad befruktning vid ofrivillig barnloshet. Stockholm, SPRI, 1990.
17. Greenfield DA, Diamond MP, DeCherney AH. Grief reactions following in vitro fertilization treatment. J Psychosom Obstet Gynecol 1988;8:169–174.
18. Baram D, Tourtelot E, Muechler E, et al. Psychosocial adjustment following unsuccessful in vitro fertilization. J Psychosom Obstet Gynecol 1988;9:181–190.
19. Leiblum SR, Kemmann E, Lane MK. The psychological concomitants of in vitro fertilization. J Psychosom Obstet Gynecol 1987;6:165–178.
20. Reading AE, Chang LC, Kerin JF. Psychological changes over the course of IVF/ET. J Reprod Infant Psychol 1989;7:95–102.
21. Reading AE, Kerin JF. Psychological aspects of providing infertility services. J Reprod Med 1989;34:861–871.

22. Williams L. It's going to work for me. Responses to failures of IVF. Birth 1988;15:153–156.
23. Bonnicksen A. Some consumer aspects of in vitro fertilization and embryo transfer. Birth 1988;15:148–152.
24. Raymond C. In vitro fertilization enters stormy adolescence as experts debate the odds. JAMA 1988;259:464–465,469.
25. Corea G. The Mother Machine. New York: Harper & Row, 1985.
26. Koch L. IVF: an irrational choice. Issues Reprod Genet Eng 1990;3: 235–422.
27. Terry P. Nightmare of high-tech rape haunts IVF programs. The Australian, 24 May, 1989.
28. Holmes HB, Tymstra T. In vitro fertilization in the Netherlands: experiences and opinions of Dutch women. J In Vitro Fertil Embryo Transfer 1987;4:116–123.
29. Yovich JL. Developmental assessment of twenty IVF infants at their first birthday. J In Vitro Fertil Embryo Transfer 1986;4:253–257.
30. Mushin DN, Spensley J, Barreda-Hanson M. In vitro fertilization children. Early psychosocial development. J In Vitro Fertil Embryo Transfer 1986;4:247–252.
31. Morin NC, Wirth FH, Johnson DH, et al. Congenital malformation and psychosocial development in children conceived by in vitro fertilization. J Pediatr 1989;115:222–227.
32. Greil AL, Porter KL, Leitko TA, et al. Why me? Theodicies of infertile women and men. Sociol Health Illness 1989;11:213–229.
33. Crowe C. "Women want it": in vitro fertilization and women's motivations for participation. Women's Studies Int Forum 1985;8:57–62.
34. Pfeffer N, Woollett A. The Experience of Infertility. London: Virago, 1983.
35. Johnston WIH, Oke K, Speirs A, et al. Patient selection for in vitro fertilization: physical and psychological aspects. Ann N Y Acad Sci 1985;442:490–503.

9

The Neonatologist's Experience of In Vitro Fertilization Risks

■

JEAN-PIERRE RELIER, MICHELE COUCHARD,
and CATHERINE HUON

In vitro fertilization and related technologies are widely available in France. Eighty-eight IVF centers are authorized by the Ministry of Public Health to provide services, but at least 80 non-authorized centers operate as well. This chapter summarizes recent data from the authorized French IVF centers[1-3] and also describes the status of IVF infants in one neonatal intensive care unit (NICU) in Paris.

OUTCOMES OF IVF PREGNANCIES

The authorized IVF centers in France performed approximately 7,000 treatment cycles in 1986[1] and 11,000 treatment cycles in 1987.[2] In 1988, 13,336 treatment cycles were reported, and approximately 10% of these treatment cycles resulted in a live birth.[3]

The rate of congenital anomalies was from 2% to 3% during each of the 3 years of the survey.[1-3] In 1988, there were 29 congenital anomalies, including 5 chromosomal disorders (3 cases of trisomy 21, 1 of trisomy 18, and 1 Klinefelter syndrome), 5 congenital heart defects, 7 genitourinary malformations, 4 digestive tract malformations, 2 strawberry angiomas, and 2 cleft lips.[3] The rate of anomalies was similar in both single and multiple pregnancies. The rate of congenital anomalies in French children from IVF pregnancies also is similar to the rates of congenital anomalies observed in spontaneous pregnancies.[4,5]

Table 9.1 shows the incidence of other suboptimal birth outcomes among IVF pregnancies as well as the expected incidence of suboptimal birth outcomes in the French population during 1988. The incidence of multiple pregnancy was increased greatly among IVF pregnancies. The incidence of both prematurity (gestational age less than 37 weeks) and intrauterine growth retardation (defined as birth weight below the fifth percentile for gestational age) among IVF births was 16% and 14%, respectively; the expected rates of prematurity and intrauterine growth retardation for the general population were 7% and 3%, respectively.[5] Most of the difference in birth outcomes was caused by the increased incidence

Table 9.1.
INCIDENCE OF SUBOPTIMAL BIRTH OUTCOMES
IN FRANCE FOR 1988

	IVF BIRTHS, %*	TOTAL BIRTHS, %†
Gestational number		
Single births	78	98
Twins	18	2
Higher order	4	0
Gestational length < 37 weeks		
Single births	10	6
Twins	34	25
Higher order	83	70
Intrauterine growth retardation		
Single births	16	3
Twins	54	25
Higher order	69	40

*Births reported by authorized IVF centers.
†Births reported among the French general population.

of multiple gestation. Even when the data were stratified according to gestational number, however, IVF single, twin, and higher-order multiple gestations still were at greater risk for both prematurity and intrauterine growth retardation compared with the general population.

Perinatal mortality among IVF births also was higher than expected. (The perinatal mortality rate in France is calculated as fetal deaths from 24 gestational weeks plus neonatal deaths up to 7 days after birth per 1,000 live births plus fetal deaths.) The perinatal mortality rate for IVF births was 17, 21, and 71 per 1,000 for single, twin, and higher order multiple pregnancies, respectively. For the general population, perinatal mortality rates of 9, 15, and 60 were reported for single, twin, and higher-order multiple pregnancies.[5]

These data suggest that the increased risk to the IVF newborn is not limited to the risks associated with multiple births. The risk of perinatal mortality is high in twins and higher-order multiple births after spontaneous pregnancy, but it is even higher for twins and higher-order multiple births following IVF.

Finally, the cesarean section rate for IVF births also was elevated. Twenty-seven percent of single IVF pregnancies were delivered by cesarean section compared with 11% of spontaneous pregnancies. For IVF twins and triplets, the cesarean section rates were 60% and 91%, respectively, while the rates for twin and triplet spontaneous pregnancies were 30% and 50%, respectively.[5]

COMPLICATIONS IN NEONATES
ADMITTED TO INTENSIVE CARE

Before 1986, very few IVF infants were hospitalized in the Port-Royal NICU, probably because the only IVF clinic in Paris was in a hospital with its own NICU. Since then, IVF services have expanded in other hospitals without NICU services; consequently, Port-Royal Hospital receives more and more transfers of premature and low-birth-weight IVF neonates.

In 1987, 25 of 350 (7%) mechanically ventilated infants in the Port-Royal NICU were from IVF pregnancies. In 1988, 29 of 383 (8%) ventilated babies were from such pregnancies, and in 1989, 71 of 423 (17%) ventilated infants were IVF babies. In the first months of 1990, between 15% and 20% of admissions to the Port-Royal NICU were IVF babies. Thus, in a 3-year period, IVF admissions to this NICU have more than doubled and now demand a significant amount of the unit's time and resources.

Table 9.2 shows an analysis of the charts of 71 IVF babies admitted to the Port-Royal NICU in 1989. This table must be

Table 9.2.
ANALYSIS OF IVF AND OTHER NEWBORNS,
PORT-ROYAL NICU, 1989

	IVF NEWBORNS *n (%)*	OTHER NEWBORNS *n (%)*
Gestational age		
< 26 weeks	5 (7)	2 (1)
26 to 31 weeks	19 (27)	104 (31)
32 to 35 weeks	43 (60)	99 (29)
36 weeks or more	4 (6)	133 (39)
Total	71 (100)	338 (100)
Birth weight		
< 1000 g	17 (24)	14 (4)
1000 to 1200 g	9 (13)	35 (10)
1201 to 1500 g	9 (13)	65 (19)
1501 g or more	36 (50)	224 (66)
Total	71 (100)	338 (100)
Intrauterine growth retardation	21 (30)	29 (9)
Complications		
Bronchopulmonary dysplasia	10 (14)	20 (6)
Digestive tract	15 (21)	44 (13)
Enteropathies	6 (8)	36 (11)
Necrotizing enterocolitis	9 (13)	8 (2)
Parenteral nutrition for more than 8 days	25 (35)	45 (13)
Periventricular hemorrhage	20 (28)	73 (22)
Leukomalakias	15 (21)	31 (11)
Survival rate	62 (87)	292 (86)

interpreted in light of the clinical disorders commonly observed in the larger population of babies admitted to the Port-Royal NICU. Furthermore, one must bear in mind that the Port-Royal NICU admits only those neonates in vital distress; therefore, this sample is biased by the strict admission criteria.

When IVF babies are compared with other neonates admitted to the Port-Royal NICU, they appear to be less severely compromised. Despite the great number of IVF infants below 1,500 g, and especially below 1,200 g, the mortality and complication rates are closer to those observed in heavier infants and not in those weighing the same. This may be caused in part by the large proportion of IVF infants with growth retardation (who are known to be less sick) as well as to their pediatric care at birth (most IVF infants were born in university hospitals).

COSTS OF NEONATAL INTENSIVE CARE

In 1989, the majority of French IVF infants (62%) stayed in the Port-Royal NICU for less than 1 month. A few (such as three full-term babies and a few infants weighing over 1,500 g) stayed for only 1 or 2 days and were rapidly transferred to level I or level II neonatal units. Over one-third of the IVF infants (38%) stayed for 1 month or longer, and of these, 10 infants stayed 1 to 2 months, 9 stayed between 2 and 3 months, 6 stayed 4 months, and 2 stayed more than 9 months. Of these final 2 infants, 1 died after 10 months from complications of prematurity, severe enteropathy, bronchopulmonary dysplasia, hydrocephalus, and terminal nosocomial infection; at this writing, the other was more than 1 year old and still in the NICU with bronchopulmonary dysplasia and stable ventricular dilatation.

The average cost of initial care for neonates with a birth weight of below 1,500 g and born in 1981 per survivor was Fr 200,000 (1981 Fr), but the cost reached Fr 336,000 in patients with bronchopulmonary dysplasia and Fr 355,000 in those with necrotizing enterocolitis discharged from the Port-Royal NICU. At that time, the daily fee was Fr 2,600. In 1990, the daily fee was Fr 6,358 or US $1,115.

Of course, the care of long-term sequelae should be added to this initial neonatal cost, especially the costs for care of pulmonary complications and neurological sequelae. These include the costs for home-care programs, rehospitalizations, physical therapy, special education, and sometimes institutionalization. When both the initial and later costs are combined, it is clear that the financial costs are great for a significant proportion of IVF infants.

PSYCHOLOGICAL CONSEQUENCES

Physicians-in-charge and a psychoanalyst conduct routine interviews of parents of IVF babies at the Port-Royal NICU. These interviews provide some indication of the immediate reactions to the birth and subsequent hospitalization of these children. In 1988 and 1989, fathers were usually quite happy; very often they were not really conscious of the potential underlying tragedy. In contrast, every mother was satisfied with finally having this most-wanted baby, but they compared their experience to a rigorous military training camp. Their initial happiness quickly turned to distress when there were several premature, sick neonates, obtained at great personal cost and often after four, five, or sometimes more attempts at IVF.

CONCLUSIONS

The neonatal risks increase in IVF pregnancies. Much of this increase is caused by the higher incidence among IVF pregnancies of multiple gestation, which is an important risk factor for low birth weight, prematurity, and perinatal mortality. Single IVF births, however, also have a higher incidence of prematurity, low birth weight, and perinatal mortality compared with the general population, so the problem is not solely one of multiple births.

The increased perinatal mortality among IVF births is well documented, but the neonatal or long-term morbidity resulting from complications of prematurity and low birth weight is not. Multiple births, low birth weight, and prematurity are risk factors for long-term central nervous system handicap, and a recent study from the United Kingdom found that multiple-birth infants were at increased risk of cerebral palsy, particularly spastic diplegia.[6] This finding is consistent with other research on extremely low-birth-weight newborns that found long-term morbidity to be the most severe in infants from multiple pregnancies.[7] That 42% of IVF babies admitted to the Port-Royal NICU in 1989 had neurological complications and 50% were of very low birth weight does not bode well for their long-term prognosis. Clearly, long-range follow-up of IVF babies is urgently needed.

Estimates of the cost to society for one IVF baby must include the cost for NICU care. Because over one-third of French NICU IVF babies remained in the NICU for over 1 month, these initial costs are high, and the long-term costs of more-frequent hospitalization and rehabilitation for handicapping conditions must be added to this. Similarly, the costs of IVF must include the drain on health service resources. If, as is the case in our NICU, close to one in every five babies is an IVF baby, then the demand on pediatric manpower and hospital facilities by the newer reproductive technologies is considerable. In addition, the psychological and social costs of these technologies to the family and the society must be included, and we know almost nothing about this type of cost. It may be greater than we realize.

At least to some extent, neonatology is rescue medicine—trying to help babies who are born too small and too soon. It has not, however, taken long to appreciate the importance of preventing these problems in the first place if at all possible. In collaboration with the obstetrics and public health specialties, neonatology has worked to prevent low birth weight, congenital anomalies, and genetic disorders and, in this way, has helped to lower perinatal mortality. Now, we suddenly find our NICU filled with high-risk newborns of our own making.

The implications of IVF for neonatal medicine previously were unclear; consequently, neonatalogists stood by while IVF clinicians in France argued that the tragedy of infertility warrants the expansion of IVF services. Today, confronted with new information regarding the risks of IVF and the increasing admissions of such babies to NICUs, the neonatologist must argue that the tragedy of perinatal death, the suffering of extremely ill neonates, and the devastation of long-term handicaps is by comparison a good deal worse.

The way in which IVF is done must be reconsidered in the light of newer information on these babies. Should the indications for IVF include (as we have found among our IVF parents) teenage mothers and mothers with children born following natural pregnancy? Should IVF clinicians be allowed to continue simultaneously transferring three or more eggs or embryos (a practice associated with the occurrence of multiple births) to improve IVF success rates? From our perspective, these practices should not continue.

Most importantly, we recommend that prospective IVF clients be informed fully regarding the immediate risk of multiple gestation as well as the long-term special problems associated with raising twins or higher-order multiple births, including such major stresses as financial worries, physical and mental exhaustion, and isolation. In addition, people suffering infertility, health policy makers, and the public must be made aware of the pediatric consequences of IVF and related technologies.

REFERENCES

1. Association FIVNAT (de Mouzon J). Dossiers FIVNAT. Paris: Centre Hospitalier de Bicetre, 1986.
2. Association FIVNAT (de Mouzon J). Dossiers FIVNAT. Paris: Centre Hospitalier de Bicetre, 1987.
3. Association FIVNAT (de Mouzon J). Dossiers FIVNAT. Paris: Centre Hospitalier de Bicetre, 1988.
4. Mortensen ML, Sever LE, Oakley GP Jr. Teratology and the epidemiology of birth defects. In: Gabbe SG, Niebyl JR, Simpson JL, eds. Obstetrics, Normal and Problem Pregnancies. New York: Churchill-Livingstone, 1986.

5. Rumeau-Rouquette C, Dumzaubrun C, Rabarison Y. Naitre en France—10 ans d'evolution. INSERM, Dion Pube., 1984.
6. Three, Four or More: A Study of Triplets and Higher Order Births. London: Ministry of Health, 1990.
7. Hoffman E, Bennett F. Birth weight less than 800 grams: changing outcomes and influences of gender and gestation number. Pediatrics 1990;86:27–34.

PART IV

LAW AND ETHICS

10

Some Legal Aspects of Modern Reproductive Technology
■

SHEILA A. M. McLEAN

To say that the legal and ethical consequences of modern reproductive technology are many and varied is an understatement. Seldom has the law been confronted with such urgent demands and such an apparent need to respond to technological change. Arguably, the need to make a statement has been given such a high profile that some fundamental questions that should take priority over consequential legal and ethical issues have been avoided, circumvented, or ignored. This chapter identifies these issues and argues that they should be addressed both seriously and systematically before considering the consequential issues emanating from this technology.

This chapter is not a review of what has happened; rather, it is an attempt to propose methods of thinking about the complex issues that arise from the application of technology to human reproduction. It considers the question of human rights in reproduction, because whether we can legitimately attribute rights may well affect the question of whether, and what kind of, legal backing is desirable or required. Whatever the conclusion on reproductive rights, the consequential issues will need to be considered, albeit possibly from a different perspective, if societies utilize reproductive technology. At this point, a brief discussion of the options open to societies is presented and questions posed about the mechanisms that might be most appropriate or functional in regulating the technology itself. Finally, issues that are important in the use of reproductive technology are considered, and principles that may be applied to achieve consistency, fairness, and non-discriminatory practices are outlined.

REPRODUCTIVE RIGHTS

It is a function of the law to both uphold and vindicate agreed-on human rights, but it is important that such rights are accepted as fundamental. Their mere assertion does not guarantee legal backing and support. As Walker noted: "It does not necessarily follow from the assertion of some right as a natural right or a human right, or as an individual or social interest, that the law will protect it and enforce legal rights and duties arising therefrom. Whether or not to recognise some interest is a policy decision for the law."[1] Claims to rights that have no legal backing or authority, therefore, are less valuable to individuals and groups than those that have such support. Equally, the assertion by individuals or groups of a special interest or "right" in respect of a given behavior implies no corresponding obligation on the government or legislature to accede to requests for facilitation or vindication of the relevant interests.

The appeal to human rights is a strong and important one, particularly in that it may require the law to offer adequate support and the appropriate mechanism for enforcement. When pressing for demands seen by consensus as fundamental to the human condition, it is now commonplace that the language of rights, whether rights are God-given or man-made, is used to bolster the claim. This chapter is not the place to engage in a discussion of the nature of human rights, but it may be important to examine whether reproductive rights have been (or currently are) recognized. If a "right to reproduce" does exist, for example, then clear consequences for societies and their laws exist as well.

This question has been examined by a number of authors[2-4] who have reached different conclusions on whether such a right exists. It is indisputably the case that when the language of rights was first applied in reproductive matters, it had a specific and somewhat limited goal. When the early feminists confronted the problems facing women during the 19th century, their translation of reproduction into a matter of rights was designed to give women the opportunity of controlling rather than expanding their reproductive capacities.[2] Recognizing that women required the status of marriage (and probably motherhood) for social and economic security, their interest was not in total reproductive or sexual freedom; rather, they were concerned with limiting the harm done to women by repeated and sometimes unwanted pregnancies. Emphasis was placed on women's capacity to limit their families by means of legal access to contraception, and then later to abortion.

During the early 20th century, the focus among these activists expanded to include the right to retain existing reproductive capacities in disputes between the police powers claimed by the government and the individual's right to self-determination—a more general right that subsumed that of not having one's bodily integrity interfered with without one's express consent to the intervention. Thus, a series of U.S. legal cases first argued the right of the government to intervene by selecting those fit for parenting[5,6] and subsequently endorsed the right of the individual to resist such intervention.[7,8] None of these cases referred to anything more than the right to freedom from intervention with existing reproductive capacities.

Ultimately, using this language of rights produced a consensus that those who could reproduce should be permitted to do so. This acceptance, however, has no consequences for those lacking the capacity to reproduce naturally; by implication, those who could not, would not. It merely restates the commitment to bodily security, self-determination, or privacy rights that generally are regarded as important by all governments. Of course, even the right to use existing capacities recently has been limited in some jurisdictions, based on a perceived lack of autonomy by those seeking to exercise it or on whose behalf the matter has been raised.[9–11]

This smacks of a return to the generally condemned eugenic approach of some countries in the early part of this century, but there seems to be some consensus that reproductive liberty should be vindicated in the majority of cases. Also, governments have begun removing some of the obstacles confronting those for whom reproduction, however much desired, was either economically or socially difficult or impossible.[12]

Modern technology, however, now permits procreation among those who do not have the existing capacity to reproduce. This places a somewhat different slant on the issue of reproductive rights, and it might well lead to different conclusions about the "right to reproduce" that also might point to the acceptability of differing responses from law and society.

The question then must be, Does it make any sense to talk of the infertile having "rights to reproduce"?[13] They may have a desire—some might even call it a need—to reproduce, but does society have any obligation to respect that by channeling technology and resources into this area? The issues of resource distribution, legal sanctions, and economic facilitation may well hinge on whether infertile people can claim such a right, but this by no means is an academic or esoteric question.

Certainly, if the "right to reproduce" is used in its historical sense, then it clearly does not and cannot include the infertile. As formulated, this right refers to the retention and use of existing capacities and not to the right to have their lack circumvented. I may have a desire to fly, but I also lack the capacity; not only would my desire be unlikely to stimulate the search at public expense for technology that would permit me to satisfy my desire, but even if the technology were available, I would not expect to be able to claim that I therefore should be able to do so and that the government facilitate this for me. This is perhaps a fanciful example, but to paraphrase the court in Skinner v. Oklahoma,[14] people may have the right to reproduce but the government is under no obligation to supply them with a sexual partner to enable them to achieve this. Reproductive technology can be seen as the modern equivalent of the sexual partner in this analogy, and both the law and society even now may well reach the same conclusion regarding their obligations to infertile people. This is not to say that we cannot reformulate any reproductive rights there may be, but so far, no successful or plausible attempt has been made to do so.

In the cause of attribution of rights, it may be useful to consider the international agreements relevant to reproduction. Thus, we might refer to Article 16 of the Universal Declaration of Human Rights,[15] which states: "Men and women of full age, without any limitation to race, nationality or religion, have the right to marry and to found a family." Subsection 3 further states: "The family is the natural and fundamental group unit of society and is entitled to protection by society and the State." We also might turn to Article 12 of the European Convention on Human Rights,[16] which states in similar terms: "Men and women of marriageable age have the right to marry and to found a family according to the national laws governing the exercise of this right."

Do these agreements not effectively give reproductive rights to all citizens, whether fertile or not? In my view, the answer must be "no." Both statements of rights are based on the capacity to enter into marriage, which in many countries—although not, for example, in Denmark—precludes those who are unable to procreate because of their sexuality. Moreover, they would exclude those with existing capacities but with sufficient handicap to deny them access to a lawful marriage. In other words, the right to "found a family"—at least as expressed in these statements—crucially depends on the right or capacity to marry.[17,18]

In addition, the right to "found a family" need imply no more than the right to avoid interference with existing capacities. In fact, both Conventions are designed quite evidently to facilitate challenges to nonconsensual intervention rather than being positive statements of "claim" or active rights. It cannot be assumed from their terminology that governments agree to do more than simply not interfere with existing capacities, and certainly none of these assertions validates a claim by infertile people that they have a "right" to reproduce.

SOCIETAL OBLIGATIONS AND PUBLIC CONSENSUS

We cannot simply revert to the days before Louise Brown (the first IVF baby), of course, and pretend that nothing has happened. Expectations have been raised. Money has been invested. Technology has been created. Whether infertile people can claim that societies should make technology available to circumvent their problems, that technology is there, is being used, and demands for access to it have considerable weight. We may not have conceded a right to infertile people, but we do appear to have accepted some kind of societal duty respecting treatment of infertility.

Not all countries have allowed the creation of a societal obligation regarding infertilty. In some countries, the costs of the new reproductive technologies are borne substantially by the government; in others, the costs of such care are borne by individuals.

One way of avoiding the problems of rights or nonrights, therefore, is to use the essentially utilitarian logic that an individual's behavior should not be condemned or controlled unless it harms others. Thus, whether or not the "rights" are available, if the technology is there and people can afford it, then we have an obligation not to interfere with their choices. In this way, the (rich) infertile would not be claiming a "right" and the government would not be acknowledging a "duty."

A number of flaws exist in this approach, however. First, it does not matter whether access is restricted to those who can or cannot pay, because even in privately funded schemes, the hidden costs impact on the community as a whole. Even if infertility treatment is privately funded and practiced, the government nonetheless has made an input in the past (e.g., through the training of the physicians who take part in the technology) and has an interest in its current application even in the private sector (e.g., as a result of the loss of skills to the public sector). Second, there is something essentially unappealing about satisfying the human needs or desires of only those who can afford to pay. In any event, if it is true that we are all making an input (even if indirectly), then an even better reason exists for refusing to countenance a system where our contribution exclusively benefits those who can afford to pay.

Consequently, it probably must be accepted that some societal response through the law is required; thus, a position has been reached where the "tail" of technology is wagging the "dog" of society. Society may conclude that no right to reproduce is attributable to infertile people and that there are more important desires that should be satisfied in a world of limited resources; however, we cannot walk away from the fact that this technology exists and that both the infertile and the sympathetic fertile know it. This raises two main questions. First, given that technology will continue to be utilized, how much should we invest in it and how will we find out what society as a whole thinks about this? Second, what principles should govern the application of the technology, and should these be legal or not?

The answer to the first question is not easy. If infertile people cannot demand duties from their fellow citizens, they nonetheless may have a claim on our humanity in the face of their difficulties. The decision about what shape that obligation takes, however, depends on consensus, and to be real, consensus depends on information. Attempting to identify a consensus, governments have adopted various approaches. In both France[19] and the state of Victoria in Australia,[20] considerable time was taken by the government to offer the opportunity for debate. In the United Kingdom and other countries, a more limited format was adopted by creating evidence-gathering committees[21] whose terms of reference (perhaps even existence) probably were something of a mystery to most of the general population.

Consensus is important, especially in societies that embrace a kind of "socialized" medicine, because in this system, the way in which public resources are used is a matter of direct concern to all. A search for consensus, however, often is a search for the impossible. Even so, the public has an interest (perhaps even a right) to accurate information about the risks, benefits, and costs of technology. Moreover, it also should have the opportunity to comment on the use of its resources.

Realistically, countries will continue to endorse and support research and practice in reproductive technology. The public input into decisions concerning reproductive technology may assist only in posing questions about the extent to which and the way in which this technology's proliferation and practice are monitored and controlled. It is technically possible that the law could declare a moratorium in the interests of stimulating informed debate and reaching a majority view, but it scarcely is plausible that any legal system would do so now. Therefore, it is important that we look for ways in which legal involvement may protect the vulnerable, enhance the interests of all citizens, and allocate resources fairly, consistently, and humanely.

LAW AND THE APPLICATION OF TECHNOLOGY

Given that no right has been conceded, that society has been informed insufficiently, and that the technology will most likely continue to be utilized, what role can or should the law play in controlling or monitoring its application? Different countries have adopted or proposed different models for reviewing the use of the new reproductive technologies. In the United Kingdom, for example, adoption of a nonstatutory, advisory model apparently worked reasonably efficiently; nevertheless, Parliament passed the Human Fertilisation and Embryology Act to establish a statutory authority to license and scrutinize practice. The actual terms of the controls exercised are substantially left to that body and were not worked out in detail at Parliamentary level.

Indeed, with the possible exception of the state of Victoria in Australia, few governments have been prepared to grasp the nettle of direct and unequivocal intervention in what often are seen as "clinical" matters. Of those that have, their attempt to do so created considerable hostility.[20] The pattern in other countries, such as New Zealand, effectively has been a policy of radical nonintervention,[22] while the government of Ontario, Canada,[23] devised a comprehensive set of guidelines.

Governments vary in their chosen method of intervention, but a relatively clear agreement exists on the issues that are of concern. Governments and their legislatures have tended to concentrate on the consequences of applying reproductive technology: embryo experimentation, sex selection, genetic manipulation, and access to technology. So far, no government has tackled head-on the question of whether the role of the law should be directive or nondirective: should regulation and control of the new technologies occur through direct legal intervention, or should it be undertaken by ethic committees or their equivalent?

In deciding this question, it may be useful to point out the folly of a piecemeal approach. Much law is created in an apparent vacuum, with little or no attention paid to its tangential consequences. Even so, the role of the law at least in part should be the search for consistency and formal justice. When dealing with one issue, it is unwise to ignore those other aspects of law or individual behavior that either directly or indirectly also will be affected.

There are many examples of the problems associated with laws that develop along set and rigid lines without taking account of their implications. In England, for example (although not in Scotland), when legislation was passed to ensure the right of children to sue for damage sustained prenatally,[24] policy considerations were used to restrict those whom the child could sue; thus, it was felt to be inappropriate that a child should be able to sue its mother, the rationale being that this would disrupt the family. While this legislation remains in place, courts in England also have been prepared to remove a child from home after birth because of the mother's behavior during the course of the pregnancy.[25] In short, the child could not sue the mother for this behavior, but the child can be taken into care because of exactly the same behavior. Which, one might ask, disrupts the family more?

Similarly, attributing rights rather than interests to developing embryoes and fetuses has profound implications for women of childbearing age. The trend in the United States of using the civil—and sometimes the criminal—law to restrict a pregnant woman's behavior[26,27] is a sad but logical conclusion of the assertion and acceptance of fetal rights. What may seem like a simple statement of faith or compassion has reverberations that can be and have been used to strike at the heart of other people's civil liberties. These are not inevitable consequences of technology itself, nor is this an argument against progress. However, if our legislatures and judiciaries are to become involved (as seems inevitable), then it is an argument in favor of looking at the whole picture before making pronouncements. Even technology designed to circumvent infertility has implications and consequences far beyond the simple desire to achieve a pregnancy.

The apparent inevitability of demand exceeding supply raises further questions. These have been largely ignored, but they affect society's aspirations to justice and fairness. For example, what of access to technology? Most advanced legal systems work (or claim to work) on a principle of nondiscrimination. In theory, this principle does more than force compliance with the evenhanded bestowing of rights and opportunities; it also attempts to offer positive choices to people, irrespective of their personal situation, unless their choice will have harmful consequences for others. Thus, if technology is available, in use, and can provide people with a means of fulfilling a much-wanted desire, then arguably it should be available without reference to potentially discriminatory characteristics. It also is clear, however, that single women, women who wish to parent without pregnancy, lesbians, homosexuals, and those thought to be otherwise "unfit" for parenting (or too poor to afford it) are discriminated against routinely in terms of access.[28]

This is justified on the basis of scarce resources and clinical judgment, as are decisions about who will or will not receive access to other technology. As always, however, these explanations remain unconvincing at the level of principle. An argument that might be convincing is one pointing to evidence that access to reproductive technology is being restricted "in the best interests" of the prospective children; if we had evidence that these groups did indeed put children at risk, then it might be agreed that such a restriction has merit. Do we have any such evidence, however? Apparently not,[29,30] but we do know that children are harmed in the standard heterosexual marriage into which we nonetheless are happy to place them. Without any real evidence that these other groups will harm the prospective children, those who manipulate the relevant technology—either with or without the direct backing of the law[31]—are in fact discriminating on the basis of societal or clinical prejudice.

Now, if there is no right to reproduce held by infertile people, this may not appear to be a problem, at least at this level. It is evident, however, that both individuals and communities are involved in the provision of infertility services (even those offered privately) by channeling skills, technology, and resources into those services. Therefore, they have some interest in the way in which resources are used and, arguably, an obligation to ensure that principles such as formal justice are upheld.

The complexities of resolving these problems might be a rationale for direct legal involvement in providing infertility services. The device of using ethics committees rather than direct law seems to be gathering increasing favor in many circles as a way of effecting some scrutiny of scientific or clinical decisions, but serious flaws exist in this approach, not the least of which is the relative difficulty of ensuring consistency of decision-making and of enforcing principles such as non-discrimination. The channels of appeal are virtually closed unless specifically legislated for.

Like it or not, most governments have become involved in legislating these matters, and the law has an obligation to eschew prejudice in favor of justice. This also might seem to argue for a directive form of legal intervention (assuming that the law addresses itself to the problems outlined here) rather than the somewhat loose framework adopted by most governments. Inevitably, this may delay resolution of the difficulties, but this may be a small price to pay.

Our current technological capacities raise many other problems as well, not the least of which are the "medicalization" of pregnancy and childbirth, the redeification of motherhood, the subtle absorption of clinical and other prejudice and (in the case of sex selection and genetic manipulation) the opportunity for cultural imperialism, demographic disaster, and a new eugenics. Ultimately, we may wish to accept these consequences, but they must be directly and unequivocally confronted before being enshrined in legislation or before the law hands responsibility over to clinicians or ethical committees.

The conclusion here must be that directive and consistent law can present a better option than the wholesale bequest of discretion to those controlling the technology. However, directive laws should be thought through completely to assess their implications for infertile people. This task can only be—and should only be—undertaken against certain principles that the law claims to hold dear (namely, justice, fairness, and nondiscrimination). The cost of applying these principles ultimately may be huge—to societies as well as individuals. If expensive technology is to be allocated on a nondiscriminatory basis, for example, then this will have serious financial consequences for governments; indeed, a whole new dilemma of resource allocation will have been created. In human terms, the availability of prenatal services, the consequences of birth, the problems of handicap, the provision of social services, the enforcement of agreements, and the status of the embryo, fetus, and child are all problems that should not be underestimated.

First, however, we must assess on what basis we are developing and offering this technology, because the consequences of that decision are of primary importance. Once this question is resolved, we can assess the kind of controls or monitoring systems that are appropriate and finally can turn our attention to the consequential problems. Unless we confront these matters—and in that order—we are unlikely to have both the logical and rational capacity to monitor or control the leviathan of progress or to assess the point at which we no longer wish to contribute either economically or societally. Without this, the law (and society) always will be "in the rear and limping."[32] Most importantly, the fundamental questions should not be begged. Before legislating or establishing ethics committees, we need to assess the underlying "good" of reproductive technology, to consider it with all its ramifications, and to decide how much, for what reasons, and in what way we will continue to invest in it. Then and only then can a fruitful legal response be developed on the basis of principle and compassion.

REFERENCES

1. Walker DM. The Law of Delict in Scotland. 2d ed., rev. Edinburgh: W. Green & Son, Ltd., 1981:9.
2. Gordon L. Woman's Body, Woman's Right. Harmondsworth: Penguin, 1977.
3. Luker K. Abortion and the Politics of Motherhood. Berkeley: University of California Press, 1984.
4. McLean SAM. The right to reproduce. In: Campbell TD, Goldberg DJA, McLean SAM, et al., eds. Human Rights: From Rhetoric to Reality. Oxford: Basil Blackwell, 1986.
5. Buck v. Bell, 274 U.S. 200 (1927).
6. North Carolina Association for Retarded Children et al. v. State of North Carolina et al., 420 F. Supp. 451 (1976).
7. Carey v. Population Services International, 431 U.S. 678 (1992).
8. Meyers D. The Human Body and the Law. Edinburgh: Edinburgh University Press, 1971.
9. Re B (a minor) Sterilisation [1987], 2 All E.R. 206 (C.A.).
10. T. v. T. & Anor (1988), 1 All E.R. 613.
11. Re "Eve" 115 DLR (3d) 283 (1986).
12. Thake v. Maurice [1984], 2 All E.R. 513.
13. Liu ANC. The Right to Reproduce and the Right to Found a Family. Aldershot: Dartmouth Publishing, 1990.
14. Skinner v. Oklahoma, 316 U.S. 535 (1972).
15. United Nations. Universal Declaration of Human Rights. U.N. Doc.A/811, 1948.
16. European Convention on Human Rights, 1950;1983.
17. McLean SAM, Campbell TD. Sterilisation. In: McLean SAM, ed. Legal Issues in Medicine. Aldershot: Gower, 1981.
18. Re D (a minor) [1976], 1 All E.R. 326.
19. Byk C. Law reform and human reproduction in France. In: McLean SAM, ed. Law Reform and Human Reproduction. Aldershot: Dartmouth, 1990.
20. Waller L. The law and infertility—the Victorian experience. In: McLean SAM, ed. Law Reform and Human Reproduction. Aldershot: Dartmouth, 1990.

21. Committee of Enquiry into Human Fertilisation and Embryology (Warnock Committee)—Report, Cmnd 9314/1984. London: HMSO, 1984.
22. Henaghan RM. Law reform and human reproduction in New Zealand. In: McLean SAM, ed. Law Reform and Human Reproduction. Aldershot: Dartmouth, 1990.
23. Dickens B. The Ontario Law Reform Commission's project on human artificial reproduction. In: McLean SAM, ed. Law Reform and Human Reproduction. Aldershot: Dartmouth, 1990.
24. Congenital Disabilities (Civil Liability) Act of 1976.
25. D. v. Berkshire C.C. [1987], 1 All E.R. 20.
26. Kolder UEB, Gallagher J, Parsons MT. Court-ordered obstetrical intervention. N Engl J Med 1987;316:1192.
27. Johnsen D. A new threat to pregnant women's autonomy. Hastings Cent Rep 1987;33:33–40.
28. Singer P, Wells D. In vitro fertilisation—the major issues. J Med Ethics 1983;9:192–199.
29. Hanscombe G. The right to lesbian parenthood. J Med Ethics 1983; 9:133–135.
30. Golumbok S, Rust J. The Warnock Report and single women: what about the children? J Med Ethics 1986;12:182–186.
31. R. v. Ethical Committee of St Mary's Hospital, Manchester. The Guardian, 28 October 1987, [1988] 1 FLR 512.
32. Windeyer J. In: Mount Isa Mines Ltd. v. Pusey (1970), 125 CLR 383, at p. 395.

11

Equity and Resource Distribution in Infertility Care

■

PER-GUNNAR SVENSSON
and PATRICIA STEPHENSON

Like many other medical technologies of dubious benefit, IVF and related technologies still have edged their way into mainstream medical practice. Ignoring the relatively low success rates, the medical community has accepted IVF as standard practice, stating its widespread availability and the seemingly high public demand for services as their rationale.

In turn, the medical community and other special-interest groups have pressured decision makers to acknowledge IVF as a bona fide therapeutic modality deserving funding under national health insurance schemes. Decision makers, however, are reluctant to do so in light of rising health care costs; moreover, they are not at all sure whether infertility services should be equated with other health care services as infertility is a social problem and not a disease.

Decision makers, therefore, are at the center of a health policy conundrum. What can be done to help infertile people? What priority should be given to infertility services (especially IVF) vis-à-vis other health services? How can scarce health care resources be distributed equitably and with maximum benefit to the public's health? We do not propose to offer easy answers to these questions; rather, in this chapter, we attempt to outline the major issues involved in decision-making for rational health policy.

DEFINING THE POPULATION

The first step toward rational planning for providing health services is to define the population needing services. A model for estimating IVF service needs follows.

This model assumes that the point prevalence of infertility derived from a cross-sectional survey of the population can be equated with the prevalence of infertility in a cohort of reproductive-aged women. This assumption can be made because infertility is not a static condition; in a female population, the pool of infertile women increases as new cases are identified and decreases as identified cases seek and achieve social and medical solutions for their infertility or age and become ineligible for services.

If we assume that the prevalence of infertility is 5%,[1] then if country X has 50,000 female births per year (a birth cohort), 2,500 will be infertile at reproductive age. If we also assume that at least half of these women will not be candidates for IVF or will choose social solutions or other medical treatments instead, then approximately 1,250 women per year will need IVF services.

The most efficient treatment capacity for an IVF clinic is 750 started treatments per year (see Chapter 6 of the present volume). If clinics offer a maximum of three treatment cycles to each woman, then approximately 325 women can be treated per clinic per year assuming a 10% success rate (live-birth pregnancy per 100 started treatments). This means that approximately four clinics of this capacity at most are needed to meet the demand for services at equilibrium.

RESOURCE DISTRIBUTION

Of course, four clinics would be the maximum number needed if country X decided to make IVF a priority health care service and to budget health care funds accordingly. In these times of budgetary cutbacks and fiscal belt-tightening, not all health care systems are either willing or able to take this step.

Some systems have attempted to set health care priorities by a rational decision-making process that takes public opinion into account. For example, in Oregon, eligibility for public health insurance funds was extended to cover all persons with incomes below the federal poverty level, but to accommodate the influx of new recipients, limits on the medical services that would be paid for through public monies had to be set. All available medical services were ranked by order of priority using both cost–utility and consensus approaches. (The cost–utility approach ranks treatments in order of benefits to the patient receiving treatment per unit cost.) The final priority list contained 714 items; IVF ranked near the bottom at number 701.[2]

Other attempts by private health insurance corporations in the United States to assess public opinion regarding health care priorities have produced similar results. A recent Harris poll of 1,250 randomly selected respondents sampled from the U.S. general population ranked IVF last in importance among 20 health services.[3]

Setting priorities for health care services involves tough choices, but the benefits are clear. Everybody has access to basic services. Services that do the most to promote the public's health are protected. All interested parties have a voice in the decision-making process, and the confusion that evolves from basing health care funding decisions on the interests of powerful, selected individuals is eliminated—or at least held in check. Health care decision makers can go beyond the question "How many clinics of what capacity are needed?" to "What is the priority for IVF in the overall system of health care services for women, adults, children and the elderly?"

EQUITY (OR THE LACK OF)

In countries with a large private health sector, the availability of IVF hinges on a couple's ability to pay.[4] "Socialized" health care systems go a long way toward eliminating inequities, but they do not succeed entirely. There usually are differences in utilizing discretionary health services along both ethnic and social class lines. Furthermore, in systems where private clinics are allowed to offer services outside the public system, special problems arise. In Sweden, for example, almost half of all IVF treatments per year are performed in private clinics.[5] In four private clinics, 1,200 treatments are performed annually, while in the eight public hospitals offering the service, 1,500 treatments are performed annually. Those who can afford to utilize private service will cut their waiting time from 4 to 8 years using the public sector to 10 months in the private sector. The physicians working in the private clinics work in the public sector, however, and state funds paid for their training and support their practices.

Few empirical studies of client socioeconomic characteristics have been published. One study of 75 couples admitted consecutively to an IVF program at Yale University Hospital[6] found a high overrepresentation of white, well-educated, middle- to upper-class couples. Only 3% had ever experienced unemployment, and no one had been fired from a job or had been in jail. Similarly, a study from Australia[7] demonstrated a clear socioeconomic bias in who receives IVF services. In a sample of 1,240 couples drawn from two private centers, the majority (54%) came from the highest socioeconomic quartile, and the "incidence rate" of enrollment of this group was 50% higher than that expected for other segments of the population. Also, males who were professionals, sales workers, or members of the armed forces had more than twice the rate of participation compared with tradesmen, production workers, and laborers. No comparison was made of the users of public clinics.

More worrisome than the passive discrimination arising from self-selection for treatment or exclusion on the basis of ability to pay are the social criteria imposed by physicians and other decision makers to determine eligibility for IVF. Providers base their policies on conventional assumptions about the ideal environment for child-rearing: the stereotype of the contemporary, white, westernized, middle-class, nuclear family.[8] Few IVF programs in the world accept lesbians or single women although many (but not all) accept unmarried couples in a "stable relationship."[9] The result is the denial of parental aspirations to those who do not conform to the norm.[8]

It is clear, however, that a clinician's (or anyone else's) ability to judge a priori "good parents" is quite limited. According to Mary Warnoch, chairperson of the United Kingdom Committee of Inquiry to investigate human IVF and embryology services, "If we do make such judgements for the sake of the child we are hard put to support them by factual evidence. We are surreptiously making moral judgements."[10]

CONCLUSIONS

Until now, discussions of IVF and infertility care generally have neglected to consider the economical constraints prevalent in most health care systems today. No health care system can afford to do everything. The key to maximizing public health in the face of these realities is to allocate health care resources (money, manpower, research funds, and so forth) according to priorities and in the most equitable manner possible. For unlimited resources to be allocated to IVF, they must be diverted from some other service, for example, hip joint replacements, cataract operations, or long-term care for the elderly. Infertility care, therefore, must be seen in the context of all available health care services and be assigned priority accounting for budgetary constraints and estimated need for services within this context.

Still, IVF and other related services should not be rationed on the basis of social prejudice. Restrictions based on social criteria are irrelevant and discriminatory. As it now stands, physicians in many countries are allowed to discriminate in the provision of IVF services in ways that the law would never tolerate if the commodity in question were housing, education or employment opportunity.[11]

Lastly, as Hull[12] pointed out, the major issue requiring resolution with respect to equity in resource allocation for the diagnosis and treatment of infertility is not how much to spend or who should foot the bill, but rather whether IVF is safe and efficacious. Until the requisite empirical information for analyzing this issue has been obtained, it would be unethical to divert resources from other medical interventions already known to be safe and efficacious.[12] For decision makers considering the place of IVF in infertility care and in health services in general, we urge a policy of rational consumption, eschewing both the temptations to condemn IVF entirely and to allow IVF services to proliferate unchecked.[13]

REFERENCES

1. Leridon H. Sterilité, hypofertilité et infecondité en France. Population 1984;4:807–836.
2. Dixon J, Welch HG. Priority setting: lessons from Oregon. Lancet 1991;i:891–894.
3. McDonald M. What to consider in covering conception. Business Health August 1989:45–54.
4. Wagner MG, St. Clair PA. Are in vitro fertilisation and embryo transfer of benefit to all? Lancet 1989;ii:1027–1038.
5. Wikland M. Organisation och tillgäanglighet av IVF i Sverige. Läkartidningen 1990;87:2967.
6. Haseltine FP. Psychological interviews in screening couples undergoing in vitro fertilization. Ann N Y Acad Sci 1985;442:504–522.
7. Webb S. In vitro fertilisation and related procedures in Western Australia, 1983–1987. Occasional paper/26. Perth: Health Dept. of Western Australia, 1988.
8. Blyth E. Assisted reproduction: what's in it for the children? Child Soc 1990;42:167–182.
9. Steptoe B. The selection of couples for in vitro fertilization. Ann N Y Acad Sci 1985;442:487–489.
10. Warnoch M. Ethics, decision-making and social policy. Community Care 1987;685:18–23.
11. St. Clair Stephenson P, Wagner MG. Turkey baster babies: a view from Europe. Milbank Q 1991;69:45–50.
12. Hull RT. Ethical Issues in the New Reproductive Technologies. Belmont, CA: Wadsworth, 1990:88–147.
13. Bonnickson L. In Vitro Fertilization: Building Policy from Laboratories to Legislature. New York: Columbia University Press, 1989.

ABOUT THE CONTRIBUTORS

H. DAVID BANTA graduated in medicine from Duke University and in public health from Harvard University. He was manager of the health program of the Office of Technology Assessment of the U.S. Congress from 1978 to 1981 and assistant director of the Office of Technology Assessment from 1981 to 1983. In 1985, he moved to the Netherlands to direct a special research project sponsored by the Dutch government and the World Health Organization on future health care technology. Since 1987, he has continued to work in the Netherlands as a World Health Organization consultant, most recently with the Netherlands Organization for Applied Scientific Research. Recently, he has directed European Community–funded projects on medical lasers and minimally invasive surgery.

DITTA BARTELS studied molecular biology at the University of Sydney and wrote her Ph.D. dissertation on the history of molecular biology. She has worked at the New South Wales Science and Technology Council and as senior lecturer in science policy at the University of New South Wales. She currently is director of European Affairs at the University of New South Wales and president of the Federation of Australian Scientific and Technological Societies. She recently returned from Europe after spending 3 years as Counselor for Industry, Science, and Technology at the Australian Embassy in Bonn.

MICHELE COUCHARD is Chargèe de Recherches of INSERM and a pediatrician. Dr. Couchard works at the Centre for Neonatal

Biological Research and Department of Neonatal Medicine, Port Royal Maternity Hospital, Paris.

GER HANN is an econometrician who worked for 6 years at the University of Limburg, the Netherlands, both in the Department of Health Economics and at the Institute for Medical Technology Assessment. His main interest is the evaluation of health care. His Ph.D. dissertation dealt with a medical, economic, and psychosocial evaluation of IVF in the Netherlands. Today, he is assistant director of the Dutch private health insurer Interpolis.

CATHERINE HUON is a pediatrician and works in the Department of Neonatal Medicine, Port Royal Maternity Hospital, Paris.

LENE KOCH holds an M.A. (Anglo-Saxon studies) and a Ph.D. (social medicine) from the University of Copenhagen. She has published numerous articles and books on women's health. She currently is studying social aspects of modern human genetics as a research fellow at the Institute for Social Medicine, University of Copenhagen.

FRANÇOISE LABORIE is a researcher at the National Centre of Scientific Research in Paris. She first trained and worked as a chemist in macromolecular chemistry, then later became a sociologist. She received her doctorate in 1967. Her fields of activity are the analyses of the social implications of science and research in general and biology in particular. Since 1985, she has been analyzing what is at stake for scientists, practitioners, and women in the development of the new reproductive technologies.

SHEILA A. M. McLEAN is the Foundation International Bar Association Professor of Law and Ethics in Medicine at Glasgow University. She also is director of the Institute of Law and Ethics in Medicine at Glasgow University and General Editor of a medicolegal series from Dartmouth Publishing.

JEAN-PIERRE RELIER is Head of the Department of Neonatal Medicine, Port Royal Maternity Hospital, Paris. He also is a professor of pediatrics at the University René Descartes, Paris.

JOSEPH SCHENKER is professor and chairman of the Department of Obstetrics and Gynecology of the Hadassah Medical Organization, Jerusalem. He is president of the Israeli Society of Obstetrics and Gynecology, the Jerusalem branch of the Israeli Medical Association. He has served as an officer of numerous national and international societies and as a member of several editorial boards of journals of obstetrics, gynecology, and human reproduction. He has over 360 publications in the fields of obstetrics, gynecology, and reproduction.

FIONA J. STANLEY graduated in medicine in Western Australia in 1970, then pursued further training in epidemiology, biostatistics, and public health both in the United Kingdom and the United States. She established the epidemiology group in maternal and child health in Perth and now directs the Western Australia Research Institute for Child Health. She also is professor of pediatrics (research) at the University of Western Australia.

PATRICIA STEPHENSON is a health services researcher/health systems analyst with a particular interest in women's health care. She received her doctorate in public health in 1986 from Johns Hopkins University and has served on the faculty of the University of Washington School of Public Health and Community Medicine, Seattle, Washington. Currently, she lives and works in Sweden, where she frequently serves as a consultant health systems analyst and directs field research projects for several international agencies.

PER-GUNNAR SVENSSON is a sociologist whose main research interest has been in the area of inequities in delivery of health services. Previously, he worked as a scientist at the World Health

Organization Regional Office for Europe and is now director of the Centre for Public Health Research in Karlstad, Sweden, and professor of public health at the Nordic School of Public Health in Gothenburg, Sweden.

MARSDEN G. WAGNER is a pediatrician with specialty training in neonatology. Following his medical training at the University of California at Los Angeles, he received a Master's degree from the University of California at Los Angeles School of Public Health. He worked as a director for maternal and child health for California and as a faculty member of the University of California at Los Angeles Schools of Medicine and Public Health, then moved to Europe to serve for 12 years as the officer for Maternal and Child Health at the World Health Organization Regional Office for Europe.

SANDRA M. WEBB studied in Australia and the United Kingdom and obtained a Master's degree in Reproductive Physiology from Cambridge University. After a variety of research and teaching positions in both Australia and the United States, she joined the Health Department of Western Australia where an evaluation of IVF in that area gained her a Ph.D. from Cambridge. Her recent work has been to assist in the development of Western Australia's IVF legislation.